ANDREW McFARLANE.

Pathogenetic and Therapeutic Aspects of Chronic Renal Failure

Pathogenetic and Therapeutic Aspects of Chronic Renal Failure

edited by

K.M. Koch
Medizinische Hochschule Hannover
Hannover, Germany

Günter Stein
Friedrich-Schiller University of Jena
Jena, Germany

Marcel Dekker, Inc.   New York · Basel · Hong Kong

ISBN: 0-8247-9894-5

The publisher offers discounts on this book when ordered in bulk quantities. For more information, write to Special Sales/Professional Marketing at the address below.

This book is printed on acid-free paper.

Marcel Dekker, Inc.
270 Madison Avenue, New York, New York 10016
http://www.dekker.com

Current printing (last digit):
10 9 8 7 6 5 4 3 2 1

PRINTED IN THE UNITED STATES OF AMERICA

Preface

This book is based on an international workshop, "Chronic Renal Failure: Pathogenetic and Therapeutic Aspects," held in Berlin in May 1996. The workshop addressed a number of issues of great relevance to our understanding of the pathophysiology of chronic renal failure, as well as to the development of new therapeutic approaches to delay its progress and treat its consequences.

The first part of the book deals with arterial hypertension, hyperlipidemia, and metabolic acidosis as factors that accelerate the progression of chronic renal failure and with the effect of dietary protein restriction as a measure to slow the advance of renal insufficiency.

The second part addresses the etiology and pathophysiology of myocardial hypertrophy in general, and especially in uremia, and the influence of the dialysis regimen on the development of myocardial hypertrophy.

The final section discusses the correction of renal anemia via treatment with recombinant human erythropoietin (rhEPO), with special emphasis on its effects on cardiac function and hypertrophy and on the function of parts of the endocrine system. Also included are an analysis of the use of rhEPO in renal-transplant patients and an overview of the problems of iron supplementation in rhEPO treatment.

We would like to express our thanks to the authors for their valuable and interesting contributions and to Boehringer Mannheim, Inc., for efficiently organizing this very informative and scientifically rewarding meeting.

K. M. Koch
Günter Stein

Contents

Contents

Contributors

Bhuwnesh Agrawal, M.D. Clinical Pharmacologist, Department TM-H, Boehringer Mannheim GmbH, Mannheim, Germany

Kerstin Amann, M.D. Department of Pathology, Ruperto Carola University, Heidelberg, Germany

B. Branger, M.D. Department of Nephrology, University Hospital, Nîmes, France

B. Ehmer, M.D. Medical Operations TM-O, Boehringer Mannheim GmbH, Mannheim, Germany

W. Franke, M.D. Clinical Research, Boehringer Mannheim GmbH, Mannheim, Germany

J. Fourcade, M.D. Department of Nephrology, University Hospital, Nîmes, France

F. John Gennari, M.D. Professor of Medicine and Director, Nephrology Unit, University of Vermont College of Medicine, Burlington, Vermont

C. Granolleras, M.D.   Department of Nephrology, University Hospital, Nîmes, France

Karl F. Hilgers, M.D.   Department of Medicine/Nephrology, University of Erlangen-Nürnberg, Nürnberg, Germany

Trond G. Jenssen, M.D., Ph.D.   Professor, Division of Nephrology, Department of Medicine, University Hospital of Tromsø, Tromsø, Norway

Saulo Klahr, M.D.   Professor and Co-Chairman, Department of Internal Medicine, Washington University School of Medicine at Barnes-Jewish Hospital, St. Louis, Missouri

K. M. L. Leunissen, M.D., Ph.D.   Department of Internal Medicine, University Hospital Maastricht, Maastricht, The Netherlands

Friedrich C. Luft, M.D.   Professor of Medicine, Franz Volhard Clinic at the Max Delbrück Center for Molecular Medicine, Humboldt University of Berlin, Berlin, Germany

A. J. Luik, M.D.   Department of Internal Medicine, St. Maartens Gasthuis, Venlo, The Netherlands

Iain C. Macdougall, B.Sc., M.D., M.R.C.P.(UK)   Consultant Nephrologist and Honorary Senior Lecturer, Renal Unit, King's College and Dulwich Hospitals, London, England

Johannes F. E. Mann, M.D.   Department of Medicine/Nephrology, Klinikum Schwabing, Munich, and University of Erlangen-Nürnberg, Nürnberg, Germany

Franz H. Messerli, M.D.   Section on Hypertensive Diseases, Department of Internal Medicine, Ochsner Clinic and Alton Ochsner Medical Foundation, New Orleans, Louisiana

Leszek Michalewicz, M.D.   Section on Hypertensive Diseases, Department of Internal Medicine, Ochsner Clinic and Alton Ochsner Medical Foundation, New Orleans, Louisiana

J. Möcks, Ph.D.   Clinical Research, Boehringer Mannheim GmbH, Mannheim, Germany

W. Motz, M.D.   Medizinische Klinik und Poliklinik B, Ernst-Moritz-Arndt-Universität Greifswald, Greifswald, Germany

N. Muirhead, M.B.Ch.B., M.D., M.R.C.P.(UK), F.R.C.P.C   Professor of Medicine, University of Western Ontario, London, Ontario, Canada

Christoph J. Olbricht, M.D.   Department of Nephrology, Medical School Hannover, Hannover, Germany

R. Oulès, M.D.   Department of Nephrology, University Hospital, Nîmes, France

O. Quarder, M.D.   Department VA-MKP, Boehringer Mannheim GmbH, Mannheim, Germany

Michael Rambausek, M.D.   Departments of Internal Medicine and Pathology, Ruperto Carola University, Heidelberg, Germany

Eberhard Ritz, M.D., Ph.D., F.R.C.P.C.   Professor of Internal Medicine, Division of Nephrology, Department of Internal Medicine, Ruperto Carola University, Heidelberg, Germany

Franz Schaefer, M.D.   Assistant Professor of Pediatrics, Division of Pediatric Nephrology, Children's Hospital and University of Heidelberg, Heidelberg, Germany

S. Scheler, M.D.   Medizinische Klinik und Poliklinik B, Ernst-Moritz-Arndt-Universität Greifswald, Greifswald, Germany

P. Scigalla, M.D.   Clinical Research, Boehringer Mannheim GmbH, Mannheim, Germany

Ute Schwarz, M.D.   Departments of Internal Medicine and Pathology, Ruperto Carola University, Heidelberg, Germany

S. Shaldon, M.D.   Department of Nephrology, University Hospital, Nîmes, France

Günter Stein, M.D.   Professor, Division of Nephrology, Department of Internal Medicine, Friedrich-Schiller University of Jena, Jena, Germany

B. E. Strauer, M.D.   Medizinische Klinik und Poliklinik B, Heinrich-Heine-Universität Düsseldorf, Düsseldorf, Germany

R. Vanholder, M.D., Ph.D.   Department of Nephrology, University Hospital, Ghent, Belgium

Birgit van Kaick, M.D.   Division of Pediatric Nephrology, Children's Hospital and University of Heidelberg, Heidelberg, Germany

W. H. M. van Kuijk, M.D., Ph.D.   Department of Internal Medicine, University Hospital Maastricht, Maastricht, The Netherlands

A. Van Loo, M.D.   Department of Nephrology, University Hospital, Ghent, Belgium

Roland Veelken, M.D.   Department of Medicine/Nephrology, University of Erlangen-Nürnberg, Nürnberg, Germany

V. Wizemann, M.D.   Internist, Nephrology, Georg-Haas-Dialysezentrum, Giessen, Germany

Isabelle Wolff, M.D.   Department of Medicine/Nephrology, Klinikum Schwabing, Munich, Germany

A. Zein, M.D.   Department of Nephrology, University Hospital, Nîmes, France

1

Relevance of Diet in the Progression of Renal Insufficiency

Saulo Klahr   Washington University School of Medicine at Barnes-Jewish Hospital, St. Louis, Missouri

INTRODUCTION

Early studies showing that patients with chronic renal insufficiency and severe uremia improved symptomatically when dietary protein was restricted provided the initial rationale for dietary therapy (1,2). Subsequently, clinical trials prompted several groups (3–8) to suggest that protein restriction was also effective in slowing the progressive loss of renal function in patients with advanced chronic renal disease—glomerular filtration rate (GFR) less than 25 ml/min.

This chapter presents the pertinent information as to whether protein restriction delays the progression of renal disease and prolongs the time to end-stage renal disease requiring replacement therapy. Besides its potential role in slowing the progression of renal disease, there are other reasons for recommending a certain degree of protein restriction in patients with far advanced renal insufficiency. Protein restriction decreases the daily intake of phosphorus and curtails the generation of hydrogen (acid), hence forestalling the development of metabolic acidosis as well as diminishing the amount of phosphate-binding drugs that must be given to prevent hyperphosphatemia and the secondary hyperparathyroidism that are commonly observed in patients with far advanced renal disease. It is known that metabolic acidosis increases protein catabolism (9). Prevention of metabolic acidosis by some degree of protein restriction may ameliorate protein degradation in patients with advanced chronic renal failure. Another benefit of a low-protein diet in patients with advanced renal insufficiency is a possible reduction in the levels of serum lipids (10), which might decrease the risk of cardiovascular disease, one of the major causes of death in such patients.

EFFECTS OF PROTEIN INTAKE ON RENAL FUNCTION

In normal individuals, the amount of protein in the diet modulates the level of renal function (11). An acute protein load increases the GFR transiently, and a sustained higher average protein intake is associated with a higher basal level of GFR. Similar—although smaller—effects are observed in patients with chronic renal disease. On the other hand, reduction in the amount of protein intake lowers basal GFR in normal humans and in patients with renal disease (12). In the past 20 years, the suggestion that dietary protein restriction might slow the progression of renal disease has been renewed, supported by the observation of a variety of physiological mechanisms that might be contributory and by strong evidence of the beneficial effects of dietary protein restriction in animals. In contrast to studies in animals with experimental renal disease, human studies have not shown an unequivocal benefit of dietary protein restriction in the progression of renal disease. Many of the human studies that reported a beneficial effect have been criticized because of flaws in design, including the lack of randomization, the use of retrospective analysis, deficiencies in the assessment of compliance, and the use of concentrations of serum creatinine or creatinine clearance to assess the changes in the rate of decline of renal function.

THE ROLE OF PROTEIN RESTRICTION
IN THE PROGRESSION OF RENAL DISEASE

The MDRD Study

A major trial, the Modification of Diet in Renal Disease (MDRD) Study, was recently completed. This study evaluated the effect of dietary protein restriction in patients with renal diseases of diverse etiology (13). Furthermore, in the last few years, at least two meta-analyses of the effects of protein restriction on the progression of renal disease have been published (14,15). The intention-to-treat analysis of the MDRD Study indicated that in patients with moderate renal insufficiency (GFR at baseline of 25–55 ml/min: patients in study A), there was a faster decline in mean GFR during the first 4 months after randomization but a slower mean decline thereafter in patients who were prescribed a low-protein diet (0.58 g/kg/day) compared to a usual protein diet (1.3 g/kg/day), but no significant difference in the level of GFR at 3 years of follow-up. A longer follow-up would have been required to demonstrate a beneficial effect from this dietary intervention in patients with moderate renal insufficiency. On the other hand, in patients with more advanced renal insufficiency (GFR levels of 13–24 ml/min: study B), there was a trend (p = 0.066) toward a slower mean decline in GFR (3.6 ml/min/year) in patients who were prescribed a very-low-protein diet supplemented with a mixture of keto acids and amino acids, compared to patients who were prescribed a low-protein diet (4.4 ml/min/year). There was, however, no significant effect on the time to renal failure or death.

The conclusion of the intention-to-treat analysis (13) was that the results did not prove a beneficial effect of the very-low-protein diet compared to the low-protein diet in the progression of renal disease in patients with advanced renal insufficiency. However, it should be noted that a usual protein diet was not included in study B. Hence, the intention-to-treat analysis did not address the question of whether either the low-protein diet or the very-low-protein diet supplemented with the keto acid–amino acid mixture slows the progression of advanced renal disease when compared to a usual diet.

In study B of the MDRD Study, the range of achieved protein intake—as opposed to prescribed intake—was wide, with some patients ingesting an amount of protein similar to that observed in study A patients assigned to the usual protein diet. Thus, correlational analyses were designed to determine whether achieved low or very low protein intake is related to the rate of loss of GFR and the progression of advanced renal disease. Two hundred fifty-five patients between the ages of 18 and 70 years and baseline GFRs of 13–24 ml/min participated in study B of the MDRD Study. Patients with diabetes requiring insulin were excluded. One of two interventions was randomly assigned to each patient: a low (0.58 g protein/ kg/day)- or a very-low (0.28 g protein/kg/day)-protein diet supplemented with keto–amino acids (0.28 g/kg/day). The main outcome was a comparison of protein intake from food or from food and supplements between diet groups and a correlation of protein intake with the rate of decline in GFR and time to renal failure or death (16).

Analysis of the groups demonstrated that total protein intake from food and supplements was lower ($p < 0.0001$) in patients randomized to the very-low-protein-diet group (0.66 g/kg/ day) than protein intake from food alone in patients randomized to the low-protein diet (0.73 g/kg/day). For correlational analysis, patients assigned to both diets were considered as one group, controlled for baseline factors associated with a faster progression of renal disease. An actual 0.2 g/kg/day lower total protein intake (including both food and supplements) was associated with a 1.1 ml/min/year slower mean decline in GFR ($p = 0.011$), equivalent to 29% of the mean GFR decline. After adjusting for achieved total protein intake, no independent effect of prescribing the keto–amino acid supplement to slow the GFR decline could be detected. The GFR decline was extrapolated to the time the patients would develop renal failure. A patient with a 29% reduction in the rate of loss of GFR would experience a 41% prolongation in the time to renal failure and hence a delay in starting renal replacement therapy. Similar analysis conducted in study B of the MDRD Study revealed a longer time to renal failure in patients with lower total protein intake. This secondary analysis of the MDRD Study (16) suggests that a lower protein intake, but not the keto–amino acid supplement, retards the rate of progression of advanced renal insufficiency. Consequently, in patients with a GFR less than 25 ml/min, it is probably indicated to prescribe dietary protein intakes of 0.6 g/kg/day.

Studies of Diabetic Nephropathy

Previous studies have also suggested that restriction of dietary protein is beneficial in patients with diverse renal diseases, including diabetic nephropathy. Zeller et al. (17) examined the effects of a reduced intake of protein and phosphorus on the progression of renal disease in patients with insulin-dependent diabetes mellitus and clear evidence of nephropathy. The experimental diet (studied in 33 patients) contained 0.6 g protein/kg ideal weight/day, 500–1000 mg phosphorus, and 2000 mg sodium. The control diet (in 35 patients) was each patient's prestudy diet, provided that it contained 2000 mg sodium and at least 1 g protein per kg/day and 1000 mg phosphorus. Renal function assessed at 3–6-month intervals included measurements of iothalamate and creatinine clearances. The patients were followed for a minimum of 1 year (mean 34.7 months). Patients who followed the study diet for a mean of 37.1 months had a decline in iothalamate clearance of 0.043 ml/sec/month and in creatinine clearance of 0.0055 ml/sec/month; values in the group ingesting 1 g protein per kg body weight were 0.0168 and 0.0135, respectively ($p < 0.005$). In this study, dietary restriction of protein and phosphorus was shown to retard the progression of renal failure in patients with type I diabetes mellitus who had nephropathy.

Walker et al. (18) examined the clinical course of 19 insulin-dependent diabetic patients who had persistent proteinuria and ate an unrestricted diet containing an average of 1.13 g protein/kg body weight/day. When the patients switched to a diet averaging 0.67 g protein/kg body weight/day, the rate of decline in GFR slowed significantly, from 0.61 to 0.4 ml/min/month. This slowing of progression was significant even after the results were adjusted for differences in blood pressure, caloric intake, and levels of glycosylated hemoglobin. Albumin excretion and its fractional clearance also decreased when the patients were switched to the low-protein diet.

Other Studies of Protein Restriction in Renal Disease of Diverse Etiology

Ihle et al. (5) conducted a prospective, randomized study of the efficacy of protein restriction in slowing the rate of progression of renal disease in patients with a variety of renal diseases. The study lasted 18 months and included 64 patients with serum creatinine levels ranging from 350 to 1000 μM per liter. The patients were randomly assigned to follow either a regular diet or an isocaloric-protein-restricted diet (0.4 g protein/kg body weight/day). Blood-pressure levels and ingestion of calcium and phosphorus were similar in the two groups. End-stage renal failure developed in nine of the 33 patients (27%) who followed the regular diet during the study as compared with two of the 31 patients (6%) who followed the protein-restricted diet ($p < 0.005$). The mean GFR, as measured by the clearance of chromium-tagged EDTA, fell from 0.25 ± 0.03 to 0.10 ± 0.05 ml/sec ($p < 0.01$) in the group on the regular diet, whereas it fell from $0.23 \pm .004$ to 0.20 ± 0.05 ml/sec (p not significant) in the group on the protein-restricted diet. The authors concluded that dietary protein restriction was effective in slowing the rate of progression of chronic renal failure of diverse etiology.

D'Amico et al. (19) recently studied 128 patients with different renal diseases and chronic renal insufficiency. They stratified the patients according to the underlying disease in a randomized controlled trial to investigate the effects on the rate of renal-function decline of two diets: a protein diet of 1 g protein/kg body weight and a low-protein diet of 0.6 g protein/kg body weight. Patients received the diets for 27.1 ± 21.8 months. Dietary compliance was assessed by a dietary questionnaire, dietary interviews, and measurement of urea excretion in 24-hour urine collections. At the end of 6 months, the actual mean protein intake was higher than expected: 1.06 ± 0.25 g/kg of body weight in the control protein diet as compared to 0.80 ± 0.21 g/kg of ideal body weight/day in the low-protein diet. Values were similar at 12 and 18 months after the onset of the study. The endpoint, defined as a decrease in creatinine clearance of 50%, was reached in 40% of the patients on the conventional protein diet and in 28.6% of those on the low-protein diet ($p = 0.0038$). Multivariate regression analysis confirmed that a control protein diet was associated with a higher risk of progression than the low-protein diet and that two additional measurements, creatinine clearance at the time of randomization and average proteinuria during the follow-up period, were significant independent risk factors for the progression of renal disease. These factors seem to be even more important than the degree of protein intake.

Meta-Analyses

Two meta-analyses of control and low-protein diets in the progression of chronic renal insufficiency have also been published (14,15). The objective of these studies was to determine whether a low-protein diet retards the progression of renal insufficiency. The study of Fouque et al. (14) was a meta-analysis of 46 trials conducted since 1975. Of these, six randomized control trials were selected. The trials were conducted in Europe ($n = 5$) and Australia ($n = 1$), between 1982 and 1991. A total of 890 patients with mild to severe chronic renal failure were followed up for at least 1 year. In this group, 450 patients were prescribed a low-protein diet and 440 a control diet. The difference in protein intake between the control diet group and the low-protein-diet group was at least 0.2 g protein/kg/day. The main outcome measured was the number of renal deaths—that is, either the need for dialysis or transplantation to ensure the survival of the patient or the actual death of the patient. The results of this meta-analysis revealed 156 renal deaths—61 in the low-protein-diet group and 95 in the control group—leading to an odds ratio of low protein to control of 0.54, with a 95% confidence interval of 0.37 to 0.79. The authors concluded that these results in a large population of patients with renal insufficiency strongly supported the effectiveness of low-protein diets in delaying the onset of end-stage renal disease requiring renal replacement therapy.

The second meta-analysis, "The Effect of Dietary Protein Restriction on the Progression of Diabetic and Non-Diabetic Renal Disease," was by Pedrini et al. (15). They searched the English-language medical literature for publications between January 1966 and December 1994 for reports that examined the effects of low-protein diets in humans with chronic renal insufficiency. There were 1413 patients in five studies of nondiabetic renal disease (with a mean follow-up time of 18 to 36 months) and 135 patients in five studies of patients with type I diabetes mellitus and nephropathy with a mean follow-up of 9–35 months. The studies included randomized control studies of patients with nondiabetic renal disease and randomized control or time-control studies of nonrandomized crossover design for patients with diabetic nephropathy. The relative risk of progression of renal disease in patients ingesting a low-protein diet was compared to the risk in patients eating a usual-protein diet, using a random effects model. In the five studies of nondiabetic renal disease, a low-protein diet significantly reduced the risk of renal failure or death (relative risk = 0.67; 95% confidence interval 0.50 to 0.89). In the five studies of insulin-dependent diabetes mellitus, a low-protein diet significantly slowed the rise in albuminuria or decline in GFR or creatinine clearance (risk ratio = 0.56; 95% confidence interval 0.44 to 0.77). Tests for heterogeneity did not disclose any significant differences in relative risk among studies of patients with either diabetic or nondiabetic renal disease. There were no significant differences between diet groups with regard to pooled mean arterial pressure (both diabetic and nondiabetic patients) or glycosylated hemoglobin levels (diabetic patients only). The authors concluded that dietary protein restriction effectively decreases the progression of both diabetic and nondiabetic renal diseases.

Assessing Dietary Compliance and Ensuring Nutritional Adequacy

The validity of the studies described above, and indeed the success of any investigation into nutritional therapy, is based on periodic assessment of dietary adequacy and compliance. Traditionally, serial changes in anthropometrics, serum transferrin, and albumin measurements have been utilized. Considered separately, each has been found to be an insensitive index of changes in nutritional status (20). Clinicians who elect to initiate nutritional therapy in patients with renal disease—and this option cannot be unequivocally recommended—should be aware of an approach that has proved to furnish a better nutritional profile. This involves using a combination of changes in body weight, anthropometric measures, and levels of serum albumin and transferrin, and interpreting these measurements in terms of a patient's dietary compliance. Compliance with the protein prescription can be assessed by measuring the 24-hour urinary excretion of urea and estimating nonurea nitrogen losses as 0.031 g nitrogen per kg of body weight (21). If the estimated and prescribed protein intakes differ by more than 25%, it is important to investigate the presence of gastrointestinal bleeding or unexpected protein catabolism. Dietary counseling should also be considered.

When defining the protein requirements of a given patient, an adequate intake of calories must also be ensured, since for a given intake of nitrogen supplemental calories improve the nitrogen balance. Subjects ingesting a limited amount of protein are at risk of catabolizing body protein if the caloric intake is inadequate (22).

CONCLUSION

The considerable evidence that dietary restriction of protein ameliorates renal disease nevertheless falls short of establishing a universally applicable cause–effect relationship. One must recognize that nutritional therapy promises at best a slower rate of progression of the renal disease, and the likelihood of success may vary with the nature and stage of the disease process involved. For the physician contemplating dietary protein restriction in renal patients, it is reasonable to consider the finding of the MDRD Study that in cases of advanced renal insufficiency (GFR values less than 25 ml/min) a diet providing 0.6 g protein/kg body weight/day may reduce the rate of loss of renal function and delay the onset of the uremic syndrome and end-stage renal disease. In cases of less advanced renal insufficiency (GFR values greater than 25 ml/min), no clear evidence is available to indicate that protein restriction slows the progression of the renal disease. If nutritional therapy is initiated, attention should always be given to the management of risk factors such as hypertension and proteinuria, which contribute to the progression of chronic renal disease. Furthermore, assessing compliance and ensuring adequate calories in the diet are of pivotal importance if nutritional therapy is to succeed.

REFERENCES

1. Giordano C. Use of exogenous and endogenous urea for protein synthesis in normal and uremic subjects. J Lab Clin Med 1963; 62:231–246.
2. Giovannetti S, Maggiore Q. A low-nitrogen diet with proteins of high biological value for severe chronic uremia. Lancet 1964; i:1000–1003.
3. Alvestrand A, Ahlberg M, Furst P, Bergström J. Clinical results of long-term treatment with a low protein diet and a new amino acid preparation in patients with chronic uremia. Clin Nephrol 1983; 19:67–73.
4. Rosman JB, Meijer S, Sluiter WJ, Ter Wee PM, Piers-Becht TP, Donker AJM. Prospective randomised trial of early dietary protein restriction in chronic renal failure. Lancet 1984; ii:1291–1295.
5. Ihle BU, Becker GJ, Whitworth JA, Charlwood RA, Kincaid-Smith PS. The effect of protein restriction on the progression of renal insufficiency. N Engl J Med 1989; 321:1773–1777.
6. Oldrizzi L, Rugiu C, Maschio G. The Verona experience on the effect of diet on progression of renal failure. Kidney Int 1989; 36:S103–S105.
7. Rosman JB, Langer K, Brandl M, Piers-Becht TPM, Van der Hem GK, Ter Wee PM, Donker AJM. Protein-restricted diets in chronic renal failure: a four-year follow-up shows limited indications. Kidney Int 1989; 36:S92–S102.
8. Mitch WE. Nephrology Forum: Dietary protein restriction in patients with chronic renal failure. Kidney Int 1991; 40:326–341.
9. Mitch WE. Metabolic acidosis stimulates protein metabolism in uremia. Miner Electrolyte Metab 1996; 22:62–65.
10. Bernard S, Fouque D, Laville M, Zech P. Effects of low protein diets supplemented with ketoacids on plasma lipids in adult chronic renal failure. Miner Electrolyte Metab 1996; 22:143–146.
11. Klahr S, Purkerson ML. Effects of dietary protein on renal function and on the progression of renal disease. Am J Clin Nutr 1988; 47:146–152.
12. Klahr S, Davis T. Changes in renal function with chronic protein-calorie malnutrition. In: Mitch W, Klahr S, eds. Nutrition and the Kidney. Boston: Little, Brown, 1988:59–79.
13. Klahr S, Levey AS, Beck GJ, Caggiula AW, Hunsicker L, Kusek JW, Striker G, the MDRD Study Group. The effects of dietary protein re-

striction and blood pressure control on the progression of chronic renal disease. N Engl J Med 1994; 330:877–884.

14. Fouque D, Laville M, Boissel JP, Chifflet R, Labeeuw M, Zech PY. Controlled low protein diets in chronic renal insufficiency: meta-analysis. Br Med J 1992; 304:216–220.

15. Pedrini MT, Levey AS, Lau J, Chalmers TC, Wang PH. The effect of dietary protein restriction on the progression of diabetic and non-diabetic renal diseases: meta-analyses. Ann Intern Med 1996; 124:627–632.

16. Levey AS, Adler S, Caggiula AW, England BK, Greene T, Hunsicker LG, Kusek JW, Rogers NL, Teshan PE. Effects of dietary protein restriction on the progression of advanced renal disease in the Modification of Diet in Renal Disease (MDRD) Study. Am J Kidney Dis 1996; 27:652–663.

17. Zeller K, Whitaker E, Sullivan L, Raskin P, Jacobson HR. Effect of restricting dietary protein on the progression of renal failure in patients with insulin dependent diabetes mellitus. N Engl J Med 1991; 324:78–84.

18. Walker JD, Bending JJ, Dodds RA, Mattock MB, Murrells TJ, Keen H, Viberti GC. Restriction of dietary protein and progression of renal failure in diabetic nephropathy. Lancet 1989; ii:1411–1415.

19. D'Amico GD, Gentile MG, Fellin G, Manna G. Cofano F. Effect of dietary protein restriction on the progression of renal failure: a prospective, randomized trial. Nephrol Dialysis Transplant 1994; 9:1590–1594.

20. Maroni BJ, Mitch WE. Nutritional therapy in renal failure. In: Seldin D, Giebisch G, eds. The Kidney: Physiology and Pathophysiology. 2nd ed. New York: Raven Press, 1992:3471–3502.

21. Maroni BJ, Steinman T, Mitch WE. A method for estimating nitrogen intake of patients with chronic renal failure. Kidney Int 1985; 27:58–65.

22. Kopple JD, Moneton FJ, Shaib JK. Effect of energy intake on nitrogen metabolism in nondialyzed patients with chronic renal failure. Kidney Int 1986; 29:734–742.

2

Hypertension in Progressive Renal Disease

Johannes F. E. Mann, Karl F. Hilgers, Roland Veelken, and Isabelle Wolff   Klinikum Schwabing, München, and University of Erlangen-Nürnberg, Nürnberg, Germany

The regulation of blood pressure (BP) and the function of the kidney are closely related. Renal disease may cause high BP and high BP may damage the kidneys, setting the scenario for a vicious circle. Nephrologists are specifically concerned about the fact that hypertension may worsen the prognosis of chronic renal disease, and may even damage previously healthy kidneys. In this chapter we review how chronically elevated, nonmalignant arterial BP may affect the natural course of chronic renal diseases.

HYPERTENSION AND THE PROGRESSION OF RENAL INSUFFICIENCY

Richard Bright (1) was probably the first person to notice that severe renal diseases are associated with changes of the cardiovascular system, e.g., left ventricular hypertrophy, which we now relate to high

BP. Bright could not measure BP but Mahomed (2) developed a device to do so and described "arterio-capillary fibrosis" of the kidney as a consequence of high BP. Volhard and Fahr (3) thought that high BP was a major cause of progressive loss of renal excretory function in chronic renal diseases. They described a positive correlation between the extent of renal histological damage in patients at autopsy and the height of BP before death.

What data have been produced in the more than 80 years since Volhard and Fahr to support or refute the concept that high BP promotes renal damage? We know that high BP is a frequent finding even at very early stages of glomerular disease. In two studies of more than 300 patients treated for various types of glomerular nephritis, hypertension was found in more than 50%, although serum creatinine was normal in most and slightly elevated in the rest of the patients (4,5).

Several retrospective, longitudinal (6,7) and cross-sectional (8) studies have provided data—within the limitations of retrospective studies—that the higher the BP, the faster renal diseases progress. Results of the largest study, which included almost 7000 patients (8), indicated that the worsening of renal function correlates with BP even within the normotensive range. Another study (7) found evidence that this observation is more evident for systolic than for diastolic BP.

Recently two prospective studies have been published. Perry et al. (9) prospectively followed about 12,000 male U.S. veterans with hypertension. Half were black, the mean age was 53, and the mean follow-up 14 years. A total of 245 developed end-stage renal disease (ESRD). Using proportional hazard modeling, the authors showed that independent risks for developing ESRD included being black (2.2 risk ratio) and having diabetes mellitus (1.8) and a history of renal and urinary tract problems (2.2). With a pretreatment systolic BP of 165–180 mm Hg, the risk ratio was 2.8; at systolic BP >180, it rose to 7.6! A myocardial infarction or congestive heart failure during follow-up increased the risk two- and fivefold, respectively. In the MRFIT Study (10), more than 330,000 men were screened. After an average follow-up of 16 years, 814 persons had reached ESRD. A strong, graded relationship between systolic and diastolic BP and

ESRD was identified that was independent of age, race, income, diabetes, serum cholesterol, and smoking. Thus, a BP of >210 mm Hg systolic and/or >120 diastolic was associated with a 22-fold risk as compared to <120 and/or <80. The association between BP at screening and ESRD was independent of baseline measurements of serum creatinine and urine protein. As in a previous retrospective study (7), the risk for ESRD was greater with elevations of systolic and with those of diastolic BP.

ANTIHYPERTENSIVE TREATMENT AND PROGRESSIVE RENAL INSUFFICIENCY

The above-cited studies are compatible with the idea that high BP shortens the life of a diseased kidney, and possibly also of some healthy kidneys. Does antihypertensive therapy slow the downhill course of chronic renal disease to ESRD? Some smaller studies have suggested that it does, especially in diabetic nephropathy. We now have data in larger cohorts of prospective studies. The Modification of Diet in Renal Disease (MDRD) Study group looked at 840 patients with chronic renal insufficiency of various origins. In 585 persons, the baseline glomerular filtration rate (GFR) was 25–55 ml/min; in 255, it was 13–24 ml/min (iothalamate clearance). All patients were randomly assigned to a goal of usual BP or low BP (5 mm Hg difference in mean arterial pressure between the two goals). The higher the achieved BP, the faster the decline in GFR over the 4 years of follow-up. The association between achieved BP and decline in GFR was nonlinear and was stronger with higher BP. Patients with proteinuria >3 g/day benefited most from a low BP, while the effect of antihypertensive therapy was less evident with lower levels of proteinuria. However, the latter patients progress rather slowly anyway, and it may conceivably take more than 4 years to appreciate the effect of drug-induced changes in BP.

Does any specific class of antihypertensive agent have an advantage in patients with renal disease? Positive data from large, prospective, double-blind studies are available only for ACE inhibitors (13,14). Appropriate studies with other agents that refute or support such advantages have not yet been reported.

In one study, over 400 patients with nephropathy of type I diabetes mellitus were followed for almost 3 years (13). Half of the patients were treated with 3×25 mg captopril per day, the other half with placebo. It was found that captopril reduced the risk for a doubling of serum creatinine during follow-up by about 50%. This reduction in risk also applied to the combined endpoint of ESRD and death. There was a slight difference in BP between the captopril- and placebo-treated groups, the significance of which depended on the parameters chosen for the statistical analysis.

In another study, almost 600 patients with renal insufficiency of various origin were observed (14). This double-blind, placebo-controlled trial—ACE Inhibition in Progressive Renal Impairment (AIPRI)—demonstrated that ACE-inhibitor treatment blunts the progression of chronic renal failure independent of etiology. The AIPRI trial employed a practical, hands-on approach. Basically, any patient with a serum creatinine concentration of 1.5–4 mg/dl was eligible for enrollment. The patients received state-of-the-art nephrological care for a 3-month run-in period, including strict control of BP. Thus, only patients with stable and documented chronic renal failure were included. Thereafter, either placebo or the ACE-inhibitor benazepril (10 mg/day) was administered for 3 years, above and beyond the patient's usual medication. Benazepril reduced the risk of a doubling of serum creatinine concentration by about 50%, compared to placebo. With almost 600 patients randomized, the AIPRI trial is one of the largest prospective long-term studies in nephrology. In accord with the MDRD study, the AIPRI study demonstrated that any trial investigating the progression of renal diseases should include several hundred patients and an observation period of at least 3 years. In studies of slowly progressive diseases, investigators should prolong this period rather than increase the number of patients.

The renal benefit of ACE inhibition was apparent in both relatively mild and moderate chronic renal failure. Notably, the data suggest that the earlier treatment is started, the greater the benefit. The advantage of benazepril was most obvious in, but not restricted to, patients with proteinuria ≥1 g/day. Patients with adult dominant polycystic kidney disease (ADPKD) appeared to be an exception. Seventeen of 64 ADPKD patients in the AIPRI trial reached the doubling-of-serum-creatinine criterion, with virtually no difference between placebo and benazepril. This negative result is disappointing, particularly since the intrarenal renin system is activated in ADPKD. However, because the numbers of ADPKD patients are small, a benefit of ACE inhibition is by no means ruled out. It is also entirely possible that interventions such as ACE inhibition may be effective in ADPKD when initiated at earlier stages of the disease. A minor portion of the benefit achieved by benazepril may be attributed to the difference in BP between the two groups. A difference in BP between ACE-inhibitor- and placebo-treated subjects has been observed in all studies in which ACE inhibition was compared to placebo. The placebo-controlled design makes such a difference almost inevitable although medications were adjusted to keep BP within the predefined range. The question of how much the BP-lowering effect contributed to the benefit of benazepril treatment in patients with declining renal function is probably less important than it may appear at first sight. The AIPRI trial included a run-in period of 3 months, with at least five visits to provide time for optimal control of BP and any other medical attention needed. In addition to such optimization, benazepril nevertheless provided an added advantage compared to placebo.

There is more than a little irony in the fact that ACE-inhibitors have turned out to exhibit nephroprotective potential, first in type I diabetic renal disease (13) and now in a generalized fashion, including for patients with various forms of chronic renal failure (14). There is still concern about the safety of ACE-inhibitors in chronic renal failure patients, particularly in those with renal artery stenosis. When benazepril treatment was begun in the AIPRI study, a slight initial increase of serum creatinine was noted (14), as in an earlier study from our group (15). However, a rapid increase in serum creatinine concentration leading to withdrawal from the AIPRI trial occurred in only three patients given benazepril. On the other hand, five patients given placebo were withdrawn from the AIPRI trial for the same reason. Thus, while acute renal failure may be induced by ACE-inhibitors, such an event is rare even under trial conditions involving several hundred patients. The same holds true for clinically relevant hyperkalemia. This complication occurred in five benazepril-treated

patients and was observed in three placebo-treated patients in the
AIPRI study. The total number of deaths was low in the AIPRI trial;
however, the absolute number was higher in the ACE-inhibitor-
treated patients than in patients given placebo. Acute cardiac events
made the difference. We cannot know whether this difference is real
or specious, since the number of patients with acute cardiac events
was low. Furthermore, the patients were not stratified according to
pre-existing cardiovascular risk, which may have been unevenly distributed between the groups. Several ACE-inhibitors have been shown
to reduce cardiac mortality in patients at risk, and possibly to lower
the rate of myocardial reinfarctions. We do not have similar mortality data for benazepril; however, surrogate endpoints indicate that
the cardiovascular effects of this long-acting ACE-inhibitor are not
different from those of other drugs of the same class.

REFERENCES

1. Bright R. Reports of Medical Cases. London: Longman, 1827.
2. Mahomed FA. On the sphygmomanometric evidence of arteriocapillary
   sclerosis. Trans Path Soc 1877; 28:394–401.
3. Volhard F, Fahr, T. Die Bright'sche Nierenkrankheit: Klinik, Pathologie
   und Atlas. Berlin: Springer, 1914.
4. Rambausek M, Rhein C, Waldherr R, Goetz R, Heidland A, Ritz E.
   Hypertension in chronic idiopathic glomerulonephritis: analysis of 311
   biopsied patients. Europ J Clin Invest 1989; 19:176–181.
5. Danielson H, Kornerup HG, Olsen J, Posborg V. Arterial hypertension
   in chronic glomerulonephritis. Clin Nephrol 1983; 19:284–291.
6. Alvestrand A, Gutierrez A, Bucht H, Bergström J. Reduction of blood
   pressure retards the progression of chronic renal failure in man. Nephrol
   Dial Transplant 1988; 3:624–632.
7. Brazy PC, Stead WW, Fitzwilliam JF. Progression of renal insufficiency:
   role of blood pressure. Kidney Int 1989; 35:670–676.
8. Tierney WM, McDonald CJ, Luft FC. Renal disease in hypertensive
   adults: effect of race and type II diabetes mellitus. Am J Kidney Dis
   1989; 12:485–493.
9. Perry HM, Miller JP, Fornoff JR. Early predictors of 15-year end-stage
   renal disease in hypertensive patients. Hypertension 1995; 25:587–594.

10. Klag MJ, Whelton PK, Randall BL, Neaton JD, Brancati FL, Ford CE, Shulman NB, Stamler J. Blood pressure and end-stage renal disease in men. N Engl J Med 1996; 334:13–18.
11. Hasslacher Ch, Ritz E, Tschöpe W, Gallasch G, Mann JFE. Hypertension in diabetes mellitus. Kidney Int 1988; 34(suppl 25):S133–S140.
12. Peterson JC, Klahr S. Blood pressure control, proteinuria, and the progression of renal disease. Ann Intern Med 1995; 123:754–762.
13. Lewis EJ, Hunsicker LC, Bain RP, Rohde RD. The effect of angiotensin-converting-enzyme inhibition on diabetic nephropathy. N Engl J Med 1993; 329:1456–1462.
14. Maschio G, Alberti D, Janin G, Locatelli F, Mann JFE, Motolese M, Ponticelli C, Ritz E, Zucchelli P. The effect of the angiotensin converting enzyme inhibitor benazepril on progression of chronic renal insufficiency. N Engl J Med 1996; 334:939–945.
15. Mann JFE, Reisch Ch, Ritz E. Use of angiotensin converting enzyme inhibitors for the preservation of renal function. Nephron 1990; 55: s38–s44.

3

The Potential Role of Lipids in the Progression of Glomerular Diseases

Christoph J. Olbricht   Medical School Hannover, Hannover, Germany

INTRODUCTION

Because hyperlipidemia is common in patients with glomerular disease, the concept has emerged that disordered lipid metabolism might contribute to kidney damage. It has become clear that numerous glomerular diseases can lead ultimately to progressive glomerulosclerosis and tubulointerstitial fibrosis. Experimental studies have provided evidence that lipids contribute to these scarring processes in animals, but there is only limited evidence to suggest that hyperlipidemia contributes to the progression of glomerular disease in humans.

EXPERIMENTAL EVIDENCE

Numerous experimental studies have shown that lipid abnormalities can initiate glomerular injury and enhance progression of established

glomerular disease. Feeding laboratory animals high-fat or choles-
terol-rich diets has been shown to cause or to aggravate hyperlipidemia, proteinuria, and glomerular structural injury (1–6). For instance,
in normal guinea pigs, a 2% dietary cholesterol supplement given
over 70 days produced elevated plasma cholesterol, an increase in
mesangial matrix, mesangial hypercellularity, and a substantial increase in the number of macrophages within the mesangium (4).

Conversely, dietary or pharmacological correction of hyperlipidemia complicating experimentally induced renal disease in rats has
been found to markedly ameliorate glomerular injury (7–12). In this
regard, hyperlipidemic obese Zucker rats given daily clofibric acid
or lovastatin had substantially less albuminuria and focal glomerulosclerosis (7,12). In experimental nephrotic syndrome produced by
puromycin aminonucleoside, it was demonstrated that HMG-CoA-
reductase inhibition or treatment with cholestyramine significantly
reduced proteinuria and ameliorated progressive glomerular injury
in association with significant reductions in serum cholesterol (10).

Mechanisms that may link hypercholesterolemia to progression
of glomerular disease include effects of lipoproteins on vascular tone,
macrophages, and mesangial cell proliferation and matrix turnover.
In rats, micropuncture studies demonstrated that hypercholesterolemia leads to afferent and efferent vasoconstriction followed by raised
intraglomerular pressure, a hemodynamic abnormality known to be
associated with the development of glomerulosclerosis (13). Potentially contributing factors to lipid-induced vascular dysfunction include a deficiency in endothelial-derived vascular relaxation (14) and
increases in thromboxane A_2 (15) and endothelin (16) associated with
hypercholesterolemia.

There is increasing evidence to suggest that macrophages play
a central role in modulating lipid-induced glomerulosclerosis (6,17).
An early influx of macrophages into the glomerulus has been demonstrated in different models of lipid-mediated glomerular injury.
Maneuvers that deplete circulating monocytes have been shown to
reduce the number of infiltrating macrophages and diminish glomerular injury (17). Macrophages can release reactive oxygen species
(ROS) and oxidize low-density lipoprotein (LDL). Oxidized LDL
can be trapped into the mesangium more efficiency and contributes

again to the recruitment of monocytes directly or through the induction of chemoattractants (18–21). The uptake of oxidized LDL and other lipoproteins by macrophages and mesangial cells stimulates the release of growth factors and cytokines, resulting in a new cycle of mesangial cell proliferation (19,21–26). In analogy to atherosclerosis, oxidized LDL had a more potent effect, and antioxidants, such as probucol, mitigated LDL-induced glomerular injury (13,19,26). The degree of mesangial cell proliferation induced by lipoproteins was significantly increased by different growth factors, and vice versa. The uptake of lipoproteins also stimulated mesangial cells to produce increased amounts of the matrix components fibronectin and collagen, probably mediated by TGF-β_1 (27). Higher concentrations of lipoproteins resulted in mesangial cell toxicity (19,21,24,26,28).

The relevance of these results—obtained mainly in cell cultures and in rats—to human pathophysiology is questionable. In humans, primarily LDL cholesterol is elevated in the nephrotic syndrome. In the rat, the bulk of plasma cholesterol is transported in the high-density lipoprotein (HDL) fraction (29), and the increase in serum cholesterol associated with the nephrotic syndrome is due mainly to increases in HDL, while LDL remains unchanged (30–32).

CLINICAL EVIDENCE IN NONDIABETIC GLOMERULAR DISEASES

Patients with rare certain lipid disorders develop glomerular injury. The deficiency of lecithin-cholesterol acyltransferase activity leads to large lipid-enriched lipoproteins, glomerular lipid deposition, and renal failure (33). The so-called lipoprotein glomerulopathy, reported from Japan (34), is characterized by the presence of increased levels of an unusual apolipoprotein E and intraglomerular lipoprotein thrombi. These syndromes indicate that unusually large and/or abnormally composed lipoproteins may contribute to renal injury.

Patients with familial hypercholesterolemia have elevated concentrations of normal LDL. The absence of renal damage in these patients suggests that additional factors are required for lipid-mediated renal injury.

Data from human renal biopsies point to a close relationship between glomerular disease and lipoproteins. Lipid-loaded foam cells and lipid deposits are common in the solidified areas of glomeruli in focal segmental sclerosis (35). These findings do not necessarily imply a significant role of lipids in the pathophysiology of glomerulosclerosis; they may simply indicate lipid accumulation in glomerular areas with sclerosis. However, in a large study of routine renal biopsies, lipid deposits were detected in glomeruli without sclerosis by light and electron microscopy in 53 of 631 biopsy specimens. Accumulation of lipids was most often observed in the mesangial matrix and the subendothelial space. The presence of lipid deposits prior to the development of sclerosis raises the possibility of a causal relationship. Unfortunately, there were no differences between patients with and without lipid deposits with regard to proteinuria, serum cholesterol, and serum creatinine (36).

Subsequent studies identified apolipoproteins, including apoB (LDL), apo(a) (Lpa), and apoE (VLDL), by means of immunofluorescent techniques in glomeruli from kidneys with different glomerular diseases (37–39). Depending on the histological diagnosis, apolipoproteins were present in 10 to 70% of the biopsies. Likewise, the LDL receptor was identified in 15 to 63% of glomeruli, in good correlation with the presence of apolipoproteins (38,39). Mesangial matrix and mesangial cells as well as glomerular epithelial cells showed positive staining. The presence and the intensity of immunofluorescence correlated with the degree of mesangial hypercellularity, glomerular sclerosis, interstitial changes, proteinuria, and hypercholesterolemia. These morphological data raise the possibility that lipoproteins may play a significant role in progressive glomerular disease.

This view is also supported by results from epidemiological studies. A strong graded relationship of higher serum cholesterol with the incidence of end-stage renal disease (ESRD) was identified in the Multiple Risk Factor Intervention Trial (40). This study included 332,544 men, with an average follow-up of 16 years. The incidence of ESRD was 23.66 per 100,000 person-years in men with serum cholesterol >240 mg% in comparison to 13.07 in men with cholesterol <200 mg%. The Helsinki Heart Study found a 20%

faster decline of renal function during the 5-year study period in subjects with an elevated ratio of LDL/HDL (>4.4) than in those with a ratio less than 3.2 (41). A comparatively small prospective study including 43 patients with chronic glomerulonephritis identified LDL cholesterol as a significant predictor of accelerated renal insufficiency during an observation time of 3 years.

Results of uncontrolled studies suggest a partial remission of glomerular disease by cholesterol-lowering therapy. In a study of seven patients with nephrotic syndrome, effective LDL-lowering therapy with the HMG-CoA-reductase inhibitor simvastatin was accompanied by a significant reduction of albuminuria from 6.2 to 2.3 g per 24 hours within 48 weeks. Serum creatinine remained unchanged (42). In another study, LDL reduction by lovastatin did not change proteinuria in nephrotic subjects. The glomerular filtration rate (GFR) significantly increased, but only in patients with an initial GFR exceeding 70 ml/min (43). The dramatic decrease in serum LDL induced by LDL apheresis was accompanied by a more than 50% reduction of proteinuria in approximately 50% of the patients with therapy-resistant nephrotic syndrome. In some patients, a significant decrease in serum creatinine occurred (44).

So far only one prospective and randomized study has evaluated the effect of lipid-lowering therapy on renal function in patients with significant proteinuria. Although a significant decrease in LDL cholesterol was achieved by simvastatin, this change was not accompanied by significant changes in proteinuria and GFR (45). Unfortunately, this study included only 23 patients and the observation time was 24 weeks. Certainly, a larger trial with a longer observation period is needed to show whether potent lipid-lowering therapy slows progression of glomerulonephritis with hypercholesterolemia.

CLINICAL EVIDENCE IN DIABETIC NEPHROPATHY

Diabetic nephropathy evolves in two stages: 1) the development of diabetes-specific glomerular injury, which is manifested clinically as an elevated excretion of albumin in urine, and 2) subsequent loss of renal function due to glomerulosclerosis. Patients with diabetes often have changes in lipid metabolism, including raised levels of LDL and VLDL and reduced HDL. In diabetic nephropathy, prominent tubular, vascular, and glomerular lipid deposits are found. These observations have led to the hypothesis that lipids may be important in the pathogenesis of progressive renal injury in diabetic patients. The prominent mesangial expansion characteristic of established diabetic nephropathy could conceivably result from a combination of hyperlipidemia and elevated glomerular pressure. This view is supported by results from several epidemiological studies, indicating that elevated cholesterol at baseline is a strong predictor of rapid loss of renal function (46–49). Treatment of hyperlipidemic diabetic patients with the HMG-CoA-reductase inhibitor pravastatin decreased albuminuria significantly (50). However, in a subsequent randomized, prospective, single-blind study, cholesterol-lowering therapy with lovastatin in diabetic patients had no significant effect on GFR and proteinuria (51). The decrease in GFR at the end of the study seemed to be greater in the placebo group, but the difference did not reach statistical significance. Hence, it is conceivable that the study time of 24 months was too short and the number of patients (16 lovastatin, 18 placebo) was too small to detect clinically relevant differences.

In summary, experimental studies in animals have provided good evidence that lipids contribute to the development and progression of glomerulosclerosis. Circumstantial evidence, results obtained in epidemiological studies, and uncontrolled therapy studies provide limited evidence to suggest that hyperlipidemia contributes to the progression of glomerular disease in humans. The prospective, randomized, placebo-controlled studies that examined the effect of a lipid-lowering therapy on progression of proteinuric glomerular disease in diabetic and nondiabetic patients did not show significant differences between treated and untreated patients. However, in both studies the observation period was too short and the number of patients probably too small to detect clinically significant differences.

In 1992, we initiated a multicenter, prospective, randomized, placebo-controlled, double-blind study to evaluate the effect of a lipid-lowering therapy with simvastatin on renal function and proteinuria in patients with biopsy-proven glomerulonephritis and prote-

inuria exceeding 3 g per 24 hours. The number of patients randomized so far is 56, and the treatment time will be 3 years. We expect
to complete the study in 1998. There is a chance that this study will
answer the question of whether lipid-lowering therapy has an effect
on the progression of glomerular diseases in humans.

REFERENCES

1. Wellmann KF, Volk BW. Renal lesions in experimental hypercholesterolemia in normal and in subdiabetic rabbits. II. Long-term studies.
   Lab Invest 1971; 24:144–155.
2. Peric-Golia L, Peric-Golia M. Aortic and renal lesions in hypercholesterolemic adult, male, virgin Sprague-Dawley rats. Atherosclerosis
   1983; 46:57–65.
3. Diamond JR, Karnovsky MJ. Exacerbation of chronic aminonucleoside nephrosis by dietary cholesterol supplementation. Kidney Int 1987;
   33:671–677.
4. Al-Shebeb T, Frohlich J, Magil AB. Glomerular disease in hperchol-
   esterolemic guinea pigs: a pathogenesis study. Kidney Int 1988; 33:
   498–507.
5. Gröne HJ, Walle I, Gröne E, Niedmann P, Thiery J, Seidel D, Helm-
   chen U. Induction of glomerulosclerosis by dietary lipids: a functional
   and morphologic study in the rat. Lab Invest 1989; 60:433–446.
6. Kasiske BL, O'Donnell MP, Schmitz PG, Kim Y, Keane WF. Renal
   injury of diet-induced hypercholesterolemia in rats. Kidney Int 1990;
   37:880–891.
7. Kasiske BL, O'Donnell MP, Cleary MP, Keane WF. Treatment of hyperlipidemia reduces glomerular injury in obese Zucker rats. Kidney
   Int 1988; 33:667–672.
8. Kasiske BL, O'Donnell MP, Garvis WJ, Keane WF. Pharmacologic
   treatment of hyperlipidemia reduces glomerular injury in rat 5/6 nephrectomy model of chronic renal failure. Circ Res 1988; 62:367–374.
9. Harris KPG, Purkerson ML, Yates J, Klahr S. Lovastatin ameliorates
   the development of glomerulosclerosis and uremia in experimental
   nephrotic syndrome. Am J Kidney Dis 1990; 15:16–23.
10. Diamond JR, Hanchak NA, McCarter MD, Karnovsky MJ. Choles-
    tyramine resin ameliorates chronic aminonucleoside nephrosis. Am J
    Clin Nutr 1990; 51:606–611.

11. Hirano T, Morohoshi T. Treatment of hyperlipidemia with probucol suppresses the development of focal and segmental glomerulosclerosis in chronic aminonucleoside nephrosis. Nephron 1992; 60:443–447.
12. O'Donnell MP, Kasiske BL, Kim Y, Schmitz PG, Keane WF. Lovastatin retards the progression of established glomerular disease in obese Zucker rats. Am J Kidney Dis 1993; 22:83–89.
13. Kaplan R, Aynedjian HS, Schlöndorff D, Bank N. Renal vasoconstriction caused by short-term cholesterol feeding is corrected by thromboxane antagonist or probucol. J Clin Invest 1990; 86:1707–1714.
14. Drexler H, Zeiher AM. Endothelial function in human coronary arteries in vivo: focus on hypercholesterolemia. Hypertension 1991; 18: II90–II99.
15. Davi G, Averna M, Catalano I, Barbagallo C, Ganci A, Notarbartolo A, Giabattoni G, Patrono C. Increased thromboxane biosynthesis in type IIa hypercholesterolemia. Circulation 1992; 85:1792–1798.
16. Bath PM, Martin JF. Serum platelet-derived growth factor and endothelin concentrations in human hypercholesterolemia. J Intern Med 1991; 230:313–317.
17. Diamond JR, Ding G, Frye J, Diamond IP. Glomerular macrophages and the mesangial proliferative response in the experimental nephrotic syndrome. Am J Pathol 1992; 141:887–891.
18. Quinn MM, Parthasarathy S, Fong LG, Steinberg D. Oxidatively modified low density lipoproteins: a potential role in recruitment and retention of monocyte/macrophages during atherogenesis. Proc Natl Acad Sci USA 1987; 84:2995–2998.
19. Coritsidis G, Rifici V, Gupta S, Rie J, Shan ZH, Neugarten J, Schlondorff D. Preferential binding of oxidized LDL to rat glomeruli in vivo and cultured mesangial cells. Kidney Int 1991; 39:858–866.
20. Satriano JA, Hora K, Shan Z, Stanley ER, Mori T, Schlondorff D. Regulation of monocyte chemoattractantprotein-1 and macrophage colony stimulating factor-1 by IFN-gamma, TNF-alpha, Ig G aggregates, and cAMP in mouse mesangial cells. J Immunol 1993; 150:1971–1978.
21. Rovin BH, Tan LC. LDL stimulates mesangial fibronectin production and chemoattractant expression. Kidney Int 1993; 43:218–225.
22. Groene HJ, Walli AK, Groene E, Krämer A, Clemens MR, Seidel D. Receptor mediated uptake of apo E and apo B rich lipoproteins by human glomerular epithelial cells. Kidney Int 1990; 37:1449–1459.
23. Wheeler DC, Persaud JW, Fernando R, Sweny P, Varghese Z, Moorhead JF. Effects of low-density lipoproteins on mesangial cell growth and viability in vitro. Nephrol Dialysis Transplant 1990; 5:185–191.

24. Keane WF, Phillips J, Kasiske BL, O'Donnell MP, Kim Y. Injurious effects of low density LDL on human mesangial cells. Kidney Int 1990; 37:509A.

25. Magil AB, Frohlich JJ, Innis SM, Steinbrecher UP. Oxidized low-density lipoprotein in experimental focal glomerulosclerosis. Kidney Int 1993; 43:1243–1250.

26. Wheeler DC, Chana RS, Topley N, Peterson MM, Davies M, Williams JD. Oxidation of low density lipoprotein by mesangial cells may promote glomerular injury. Kidney Int 1994; 45:1628–1636.

27. Ding GH, Pesekdiamond I, Diamond JR. Cholesterol, macrophages and gene expression of TGF-beta-1 and fibronectin during fibrosis. Am J Physiol 1993; 264:F577–F584.

28. Gupta S, Rifici V, Crowley S, Brownlee M, Zihe S, Schlondorff D. Interaction of LDL with mesangial cells and matrix. Kidney Int 1992; 41:1161–1169.

29. Chapman MJ. Comparative analysis of mammalian plasma lipoproteins. II. Colowick SP, Kaplan NO, ed. Methods in Enzymology. Vol 128. New York: Academic Press, 1986:70–143.

30. Calandra S, Tarugi P, Ghisellini M, Gherardi E. Plasma and urine lipoproteins during the development of nephrotic syndrome induced in the rat by adriamycin. Exp Molec Biol 1983; 39:282–299.

31. Marshall JF. Apostolopoulos JJ, Brack CM, Howlett GJ. Regulation of apolipoprotein gene expression and plasma high-density lipoprotein composition in experimental nephrosis. Biochim Biophys Acta 1990; 1042:271–279.

32. Goor HV, Horst MLC, Atmosoerodjo J, Joles JA, Tol Av, Grond J. Renal apolipoproteins in nephrotic rats. Am J Pathol 1993; 142:1804–1812.

33. Norum KR, Gjone E, Glomset JA. Familial lecithin: cholesterol acyltransferase deficiency, including fish eye disease. In: Scriver CR, Baudet AL, Sly WS, Valle D, eds. The Metabolic Basis of Inherited Disease. New York: McGraw-Hill, 1989:1181–1194.

34. Oikawa S, Suzuki N, Sakuma E, Saito T, Namai K, Fuji Y, Toyota T. Abnormal lipoprotein and apolipoprotein pattern in lipoprotein glomerulopathy. Am J Kidney Dis 1991; 18:553–558.

35. Heptinstall RH. The nephrotic syndrome. In: Heptinstall RH, ed. Pathology of the Kidney. 3rd ed. Boston: Little, Brown, 1983:637.

36. Lee HS, Lee JS, Koh HI, Ko KW. Intraglomerular lipid deposition in routine biopsies. Clin Nephrol 1991; 36:67–75.

37. Sato H, Suzuki S, Kobayashi H, Ogino S, Inomata A, Arakawa M. Immunohistological localization of apolipoproteins in the glomeruli in

renal disease: specifically apoB and apoE. Clin Nephrol 1991; 36:127–133.

38. Sato H, Suzuki S, Ueno M, Shimada H, Karasawa R, Nishi SI, Arakawa M. Localization of apolipoprotein(a) and B-100 in various renal diseases. Kidney Int 1993; 43:430–435.

39. Takemura T, Yoshioka K, Aya N, Murukami K, Matumoto A, Itakura H, Kodama T, Suzuki H, Maki S. Apolipoproteins and lipoprotein receptors in glomeruli in human kidney diseases. Kidney Int 1993; 43: 918–927.

40. Klag MJ, Whelton PK, Randall B, Neaton J, Brancati FL, Stanler J. Serum cholesterol and ESRD incidence in men screened for MRFIT (abstr). J Am Soc Nephrol 1995; 6:393.

41. Mänttäri M, Tiula E, Alikoski T, Manninen V. Effects of hypertension and dyslipidemia on the decline in renal function. Hypertension 1995; 26:670–675.

42. Rabelink AJ, Hené RJ, Erkelenz DW, Joles JA, Koomans HA. Partial remission of nephrotic syndrome in patients on long-term simvastatin. Lancet 1990; 335:1045–1046.

43. Chan PCK, Robinson JD, Yeung WC, Cheng KP, Yeung HWD, Tsang MTS. Lovastatin in glomerulonephritis patients with hyperlipidemia and heavy proteinuria. Nephrol Dialysis Transplant 1992; 7:93–99.

44. Muso E, Yashhiro M, Matsushima M, Yoshida H, Sawanishi K, Sasayama S. Does LDL-apheresis in steroid resistant nephrotic syndrome affect prognosis? Nephrol Dialysis Transplant 1994; 9:257–264.

45. Thomas ME, Harris KPG, Ramaswamy C, Hattersley JM, Wheeler DC, Varghese Z, Williams JD, Walls J, Moorhead JF. Simvastatin therapy for hypercholesterolemic patients with nephrotic syndrome or significant proteinuria. Kidney Int 1993; 44:1124–1129.

46. Mulec H, Johnson SAA, Björck S. Relation between serum cholesterol and diabetic nephropathy. Lancet 1990; 335:1537–1538.

47. Hommel E, Andersen P, Gall MA. Plasma lipoproteins and renal function during simvastatin treatment in diabetic nephropathy. Diabetologia 1992; 35:447–451.

48. Hasslacher C, Bosted-Kiesel A, Kempe HP, Wahl P. Effect of metabolic factors and blood pressure on kidney function in proteinuric Typ 2 (non-insulin-dependent) diabetic patients. Diabetologia 1993; 36:1051–1056.

49. Krolewski AS, Warram JH, Christlieb AR. Hypercholesterolemia-A determinant of renal function loss and deaths in IDDM patients with nephropathy. Kidney Int 1994; 45(suppl):S-125–S-131.

50. Shoji T, Nishizawa Y, Toyokawa A, Kawagishi T, Okuno Y, Morii H. Decreased albuminuria by pravastatin in hyperlipidemic diabeties. Nephron 1991; 59:664–665.
51. Lam KSL, Cheng IKP, Pang RWC. Cholesterol-lowering therapy may retard the progression of diabetic nephropathy. Diabetologie 1995; 38: 604–609.

4

Is Metabolic Acidosis a Risk Factor in the Progression of Renal Insufficiency?

F. John Gennari   University of Vermont College of Medicine, Burlington, Vermont

INTRODUCTION

Metabolic acidosis, defined as a reduction in both the pH and the bicarbonate concentration ($[HCO_3^-]$) of the body fluids, is an almost inevitable consequence of chronic renal insufficiency. Measurements in patients with only mild to moderate renal impairment (glomerular filtration rate of approximately 20–50 ml/min) demonstrate an average reduction in serum $[HCO_3^-]$ of 6 mEq/L (1). Although serum $[HCO_3^-]$ varies considerably in patients with more advanced renal insufficiency, the vast majority have an even greater reduction in serum $[HCO_3^-]$ (2–4). The metabolic acidosis of renal insufficiency is due primarily to a limitation in ammonium synthesis and excretion (2). As a result, patients with renal insufficiency are unable to respond to increase in acid production with matched increases in acid excretion. In the steady state, daily retention of some acid probably occurs, although this point is debated (see later). In addition to impaired acid excretion, patients with renal insufficiency may have impaired bicarbonate reabsorption, manifested by a failure to conserve administered bicarbonate (2).

In theory, the sustained metabolic acidosis of chronic renal insufficiency could injure the kidney through several mechanisms (Figure 1). First, it is known that metabolic acidosis promotes calcium release from bones, at least in the short term (5). This calcium is carried to the kidneys and excreted, and could contribute to renal injury by cellular deposition (6). Second, metabolic acidosis is known to induce renal hypertrophy (7–10). Acidosis-induced renal growth could be a facilitating factor for mesangial proliferation, glomerulosclerosis, and tubulointerstitial injury (11). Third, it has been proposed that the increase in ammonium production and secretion per nephron that occurs with metabolic acidosis stimulates complement release, leading to complement-induced renal injury (12,13). Finally,

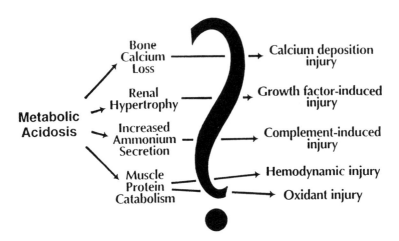

Figure 1 (Left) effects of metabolic acidosis on body metabolism and (right) hypothetical mechanisms by which these effects could damage the kidney in patients with renal insufficiency. The question mark signifies that there is no conclusive proof that these hypothetical mechanisms actually accelerate renal injury.

metabolic acidosis promotes protein catabolism in muscle cells (3, 14), and this protein catabolism could promote glomerular capillary hypertension in renal insufficiency just as ingestion and metabolic breakdown of protein do (15,16). Alternatively, protein catabolism could injure the kidney by increasing renal oxidative work, promoting oxidant injury (17). In this review, I focus on the experimental evidence for and against these theoretical injurious effects of metabolic acidosis.

CALCIUM IMBALANCE

Disordered calcium homeostasis, leading to intrarenal calcium deposition, is a characteristic feature of chronic renal insufficiency. The calcium content of the kidney is increased both in experimental models of renal failure and in patients with renal disease (6,18). Calcium deposition in the kidney has been shown to be associated with morphological mitochondrial damage and dysfunction, and has been implicated to alter glomerular hemodynamics, stimulate cytokine release, and promote renal ischemic injury (6). Cellular calcium accumulation can be prevented by dietary phosphate restriction or parathyroidectomy, suggesting that hypersecretion of parathyroid hormone is responsible, but a contributing role for metabolic acidosis cannot be excluded. Calcium release from bone is stimulated by an acid pH, and bone calcium salts are known to contribute to the buffering of retained acid (5,19,20). It is intriguing that renal calcium content is highest in patients with chronic renal insufficiency due to analgesic nephropathy, a disorder known to be associated with a larger reduction in serum [HCO_3^-] than other forms of renal disease (18). The evidence that metabolic acidosis contributes importantly to bone calcium release in chronic renal insufficiency, however, is not well established.

In a classic series of experiments in humans, Lemann, Lennon, and coworkers (4,21) showed that patients with chronic renal insufficiency are in positive acid balance. Because serum [HCO_3^-] did not change over time in these patients, these investigators proposed that the retained acid was continuously being buffered by calcium salts released from bone. In support of this theory, they produced metabolic acidosis in normal volunteers by ammonium-chloride feeding, and demonstrated that they were indeed in negative calcium balance over a period of 2 weeks (5). Moreover, the amount of calcium lost closely approximated the amount of H^+ retained. Short-term administration of ammonium chloride in normal subjects, however, is not a good model of the sustained acidosis of renal insufficiency. In contrast to normal individuals fed ammonium chloride, patients with renal insufficiency–associated metabolic acidosis have only a very minor degree of negative calcium balance (4). Correction of the acidosis in these patients improved calcium balance slightly, but no close correlation between acid retention and calcium loss was present.

A problem with the concept that bone calcium salts continually buffer retained H^+ is that the supply of calcium (and its associated anions) is simply insufficient to buffer the total amount of H^+ estimated to be retained over the many years before end-stage renal disease develops (22). An alternative explanation is that acid retention does not occur continuously in patients with chronic renal disease. The studies demonstrating a small but significant positive acid balance in these patients, however, are quite reproducible (4,21,23), and one would therefore have to propose either that a systematic error exists in these studies or that a component of acid excretion is not measured. Nonetheless, the clear correlation between acid retention and renal calcium loss in short-term metabolic acidosis is very different from the minor change in calcium balance seen in patients with chronic renal insufficiency (4,5). The latter could be simply a reflection of vitamin D deficiency, and unrelated to metabolic acidosis.

A major argument against the role of acidosis-induced renal calcium deposition as a significant cause of renal failure is the experiment in nature of type I renal tubular acidosis (RTA). Renal failure is a rare complication of this disorder despite long-term metabolic acidosis and nephrocalcinosis. In one study, creatinine clearance was higher in the RTA patients with nephrocalcinosis than in those without (24). Intrarenal calcium deposition may contribute to renal injury in patients with chronic renal insufficiency, but the evidence suggests that its cause is secondary hyperparathyroidism rather than metabolic acidosis.

RENAL HYPERTROPHY

Induction of metabolic acidosis in experimental animals causes renal hypertrophy (7–10). Hypertrophy is thought to be initiated by stimulation of transport processes within the kidney (most notably, Na^+/H^+ exchange), and stimulation of ammonium production and secretion (25,26). Although hypertrophy is an adaptive response in the short run, the renal growth response has been implicated to initiate a destructive cycle that eventually leads to glomerulosclerosis and tubulointerstitial injury (11).

The potentially injurious role of acidosis-induced renal hypertrophy has been assessed experimentally both in normal rats and in rats with renal insufficiency induced by partial renal ablation (10). In normal rats, metabolic acidosis was induced by HCl-feeding for 15 weeks. The rats developed transient proteinuria, but this abated completely by the end of the study. Renal hypertrophy developed, but histological examination of the kidneys showed no evidence of glomerular or tubular damage. In rats with partial renal ablation, correction of metabolic acidosis by administration of alkali for 25 weeks had no effect on renal size or on the degree of proteinuria, glomerulosclerosis, or tubulointerstitial damage (10). From these observations, it appears that the hypertrophy induced by prolonged metabolic acidosis is not injurious to the normal kidney, and, in the remnant kidney model of renal insufficiency, no contribution of metabolic acidosis to hypertrophy or renal damage occurs. The results in remnant kidney rats, however, differ notably from those of an earlier study of similar experimental design (12). In that study, correction of acidosis (for only 4–6 weeks after partial renal ablation) reduced both proteinuria and tubulointerstitial injury (Table 1) (12). The role of hypertrophy was not assessed in the latter study because another acidosis-induced factor was proposed to cause the renal injury (see below).

STIMULATION OF AMMONIUM SECRETION

Nath and coworkers (12,13) have proposed that the increase in ammonium secretion per nephron in renal insufficiency may cause renal

Table 1 Effect of Correction of Metabolic Acidosis on Renal Function and Morphology in the Remnant Kidney Model of Renal Insufficiency in the Rat

Study	Duration (wks)	Treatment	GFR	Proteinuria	Pathology	Survival
Nath et al., 1985 (12)	4–6	NaHCO₃ vs. NaCl	No effect	↓ 46%	↓ Tubular diameter ↓ Casts ↓ Interstitial infiltration	No effect
Throssell et al., 1995 (10)	25	NaHCO₃ vs. NaCl	No effect	No effect	No effect (far advanced injury)	No effect

injury not only by stimulating growth factors, but also by activating complement. The free base ammonia is apparently capable of disrupting a thiolester bond in the third component of complement (C3), yielding an amidated C3. Amidated C3 stimulates the alternative complement pathway, generating the chemoattractants C3a and C5a and fostering assembly of the cytolytic membrane attack complex. To test their hypothesis, Nath et al. studied complement deposition in the tubules and interstitium of rats with renal insufficiency induced by partial renal ablation (12). In a careful study using pair feeding, they corrected metabolic acidosis by substituting sodium bicarbonate for sodium chloride in one group of remnant kidney rats and demonstrated a marked reduction in complement deposition—and less tubulointerstitial injury (Table 1)—as compared to a control group given an equivalent amount of sodium chloride. To demonstrate a role for complement activation as opposed to renal hypertrophy in producing the renal injury, they induced renal insufficiency in mice deficient in C5, and showed that these rats had less proteinuria (after 30 weeks) than a control group of mice with renal insufficiency and an intact complement system.

Despite these extensive studies, the role of metabolic acidosis, per se, in stimulating complement-induced tubulointerstitial damage remains circumstantial. The high NaCl intake of the control animals, for example, could have induced injury. Blood pressures were not measured in the rats during the course of the study. The bicarbonate-supplemented rats actually developed mild metabolic alkalosis (serum [HCO_3^-] 31 mEq/L), which may influence complement activation and renal injury. Finally, the rats were studied for only 4–6 weeks after renal ablation. In a much longer study in which blood pressures and protein excretion were measured, no effect of acidosis on renal injury could be demonstrated (10). Thus, the evidence in support of acidosis-stimulated complement activation and accelerated renal damage is limited.

EFFECTS OF PROTEIN CATABOLISM

Numerous studies in humans and experimental animals have shown that metabolic acidosis stimulates muscle protein catabolism (3,14, 27–29). Acidosis-induced muscle protein breakdown is associated with increased rates of branched-chain amino acid oxidation (3,14). This catabolic process is directly attributable to metabolic acidosis as opposed to other effects of chronic renal insufficiency (27). In the short term, muscle protein catabolism is thought to be an adaptive response to acidosis, providing substrate for glutamine synthesis, the product needed to supply ammonium to the kidney. The catabolic response to metabolic acidosis is associated with an increase in glucocorticoid secretion, and it appears that glucocorticoids are necessary for the catabolic response to occur (14,29).

The protein catabolic effects of metabolic acidosis could injure the kidney through two separate pathways (Figure 1), both involving increases in "renal work." The first is by increasing glomerular capillary hydrostatic pressure, as occurs after ingestion of a protein meal (15,16). In animal models of chronic renal insufficiency, glomerular capillary pressure is increased; this increase is well recognized to be maladaptive, leading to glomerular hypertrophy and sclerosis (11). The increase in glomerular pressure is dependent in part on the level of protein intake. Reducing dietary protein intake reduces glomerular pressures and slows the progression of renal damage (15). Of note, protein restriction also partially corrects the metabolic acidosis present in the remnant kidney model of renal insufficiency (30). One can speculate that acidosis-induced catabolism of endogenous protein stores induces the same effect on glomerular hemodynamics that continued high protein intake does. Correction of metabolic acidosis in the remnant kidney rat model of renal insufficiency without changing protein intake, however, has no effect on glomerular capillary pressure (12).

The second pathway by which protein catabolism may injure the kidney is by producing "hypermetabolism" and oxidant injury (17,31–33). Morphological studies of the remnant kidney model of renal failure, as well as in humans with renal insufficiency, suggest that tubulointerstitial damage is a better correlate of renal survival than is glomerular damage (12). Harris and coworkers (17) demonstrated that oxygen consumption factored by nephron number is increased threefold in the remnant kidney model of renal failure. Based on this observation, they postulated that oxidant injury, caused by increased production of free oxygen radicals secondary to hypermetabolism, contributes significantly to tubulointerstitial damage in renal insufficiency. These investigators then studied the effect on oxygen consumption of maneuvers known to reduce renal damage, including dietary protein or phosphate restriction and verapamil administration, and showed that each of these maneuvers also decreased oxygen consumption (31,32).

Despite these extensive studies, no causative link between renal oxygen consumption and renal injury has been established. Moreover, questions have arisen concerning whether the nephron is the appropriate metabolic unit to factor oxygen consumption in the remnant kidney. If one factors oxygen consumption by gram of renal tissue, it is no different from normal and thus there is no hypermetabolism (34). Because a larger fraction of oxygen consumption in the remnant kidney is not directed at sodium reabsorption (as compared to the normal kidney), one can make the case that the increased oxidative work is not the result of hyperfiltration but is a normal requirement for maintenance of cellular integrity in the hypertrophied cells. Measurements to assess the metabolic products produced by free oxygen radical damage, moreover, do not support the view that oxidant injury is increased (33). Thus, it is debatable that renal oxygen consumption is increased in the remnant kidney, and there is little evidence that oxidant injury is occurring. There is no information concerning whether correction of metabolic acidosis in this setting alters renal oxygen consumption.

SUMMARY AND CONCLUSIONS

Despite the multiple ways in which metabolic acidosis can, in theory, damage the already injured kidney, there is little empirical evidence to support aggressive correction of metabolic acidosis as a tool to slow the progression of renal disease. Only two studies have directly addressed the role of metabolic acidosis in accelerating renal injury. Both studies were carried out in the remnant kidney model of renal failure in the rat, and, in both, acidosis was corrected by $NaHCO_3^-$ administration (10,12). As shown in Table 1, these two studies show strikingly divergent results. In the first study, proteinuria was reduced by alkali administration, whereas in the second there was no effect on proteinuria. The first study showed that correction of acidosis ameliorated tubulointerstitial damage; the second showed no amelioration. There is no complete explanation for the difference in results, but these divergent findings weaken the case for a specific role for metabolic acidosis in producing renal injury.

The most direct way to examine whether metabolic acidosis can accelerate renal damage is to carry out a clinical trial in which patients with mild to moderate renal insufficiency are randomized to correction of metabolic acidosis or no alkali treatment, and the rate of progression and severity of proteinuria assessed. Such a trial is unlikely to be undertaken, however, because most physicians agree that patients with serum [HCO_3^-] less than 15–16 mEq/L need alkali replacement, and some already advocate full correction of hypobicarbonatemia in all patients with renal insufficiency (19,20). In addition, it may be difficult in such a trial to control adequately for other factors known to influence the rate of progression. Perhaps we should rely on the experiment in nature of renal tubular acidosis. There is little evidence that the sustained metabolic acidosis characteristic of either type I or type II RTA is associated with progressive renal injury and renal failure. Although there are many reasons to try to correct metabolic acidosis in patients with renal insufficiency, slowing the progression of their renal disease does not seem to be one of them.

REFERENCES

1. Widmer B, Gerhardt RE, Harrington JT, Cohen JJ. Serum electrolyte and acid base composition: the influence of graded degrees of chronic renal failure. Arch Intern Med 1979; 139:1099–1102.
2. Schwartz WB, Hall PW, Hays RM, Relman AS. On the mechanism of acidosis in chronic renal disease. J Clin Invest 1959; 38:39–52.
3. Reaich D, Channon SM, Schrimgeour CM, Daley SE, Wilkinson R, Goodship THJ. Correction of acidosis in humans with CRF decreases protein degradation and amino acid oxidation. Am J Physiol 1993; 265: E230–E235.
4. Litzow JR, Lemann J, Lennon EJ. The effect of treatment of acidosis on calcium balance in patients with chronic azotemic renal disease. J Clin Invest 1967; 46:280–286.
5. Lemann J, Litzow JR, Lennon EJ. The effect of chronic acid loads in normal man: further evidence for the participation of bone mineral in the defense against chronic metabolic acidosis. J Clin Invest 1966; 45: 1608–1614.
6. Kramer HJ, Meyer-Lehnert H, Mohaupt M. Role of calcium in the progression of renal disease: experimental evidence. Kidney Int 1992; 41(suppl 36):S2–S7.
7. Santella RN, Gennari FJ, Maddox DA. Metabolic acidosis stimulates bicarbonate reabsorption in the early proximal tubule. Am J Physiol 1989; 257:F35–F42.
8. Lotspeich WD. Renal hypertrophy in metabolic acidosis and its relation to ammonia excretion. Am J Physiol 1965; 208:1138–1142.
9. Halliburton IW, Thomson RY. The effect of diet and of unilateral nephrectomy on the composition of the kidney. Cancer Res 1967; 27: 1632–1638.
10. Throssell D, Brown J, Harris KPG, Walls J. Metabolic acidosis does not contribute to chronic renal injury in the rat. Clin Sci 1995; 89:643–650.

11. Hostetter TH. Progression of renal disease and renal hypertrophy. Annu Rev Physiol 1995; 57:263–278.
12. Nath KA, Hostetter MK, Hostetter TH. Pathophysiology of chronic tubulo-interstitial disease in rats: interactions of dietary acid load, ammonia, and complement component C3. J Clin Invest 1985; 76:667–675.
13. Nath KA, Hostetter MK, Hostetter TH. Increased ammoniagenesis as a determinant of progressive renal injury. Am J Kid Dis 1991; 17:654–657.
14. May RC, Bailey JL, Mitch WE, Masud T, England BK. Glucocorticoids and acidosis stimulate protein and amino acid catabolism in vivo. Kidney Int 1996; 49:679–683.
15. Hostetter TH, Olson JL, Rennke HG, Venkatachalam MA, Brenner BM. Hyperfiltration in remnant nephrons: a potentially adverse response to renal ablation. Am J Physiol 1981; 241:F85–F93.
16. Brenner BM, Myer TW, Hostetter TH. Dietary protein and the progressive nature of kidney disease: the role of hemodynamically mediated glomerular injury in the pathogenesis of progressive glomerulosclerosis in aging, renal ablation and intrinsic renal disease. N Engl J Med 1982; 307:652–659.
17. Harris DCH, Chan L, Schrier RW. Remnant kidney hypermetabolism and progression of chronic renal failure. Am J Physiol 1988; 254:F267–F276.
18. Ibels LS, Alfrey AC, Huffer WE, Craswell PW, Weil R. Calcification in end-stage kidneys. Am J Med 1981; 71:33–37.
19. Bushinsky DA. The contribution of acidosis to renal osteodystrophy. Kidney Int 1995; 47:1816–1832.
20. Kraut JA. The role of metabolic acidosis in the pathogenesis of renal osteodystrophy. Adv Renal Replacement Ther 1995; 2:40–51.
21. Goodman AD, Lemann J, Lennon EJ, Relman AS. Production, excretion, and net balance of fixed acid in patients with renal acidosis. J Clin Invest 1965; 44:495–506.
22. Oh MS. Irrelevance of bone buffering to acid-base homeostasis in chronic metabolic acidosis. Nephron 1991; 59:7–10.
23. Uribarri J, Douyon H, Oh MS. A re-evaluation of the urinary parameters of acid production and excretion in patients with chronic renal acidosis. Kidney Int 1995; 47:624–627.
24. Caruana RJ, Buckalew VM. The syndrome of distal (type 1) renal tubular acidosis: clinical and laboratory findings in 58 cases. Medicine 1988; 67:84–98.

25. Fine L. The biology of renal hypertrophy. Kidney Int 1986; 29:619–634.
26. Golchini K, Norman J, Bohman R, Kurtz I. Induction of hypertrophy in cultured proximal tubule cells by extracellular NH_4Cl. J Clin Invest 1989; 84:1767–1779.
27. May RC, Kelly RA, Mitch WE. Mechanisms for defects in muscle protein metabolism in rats with chronic uremia: influence of metabolic acidosis. J Clin Invest 1987; 79:1099–1103.
28. Papadoyannakis NJ, Stefanidis CJ, McGeown M. The effect of the correction of metabolic acidosis on nitrogen and potassium balance of patients with chronic renal failure. Am J Clin Nutr 1984; 40:623–627.
29. May RC, Kelly RA, Mitch WE. Metabolic acidosis stimulates protein degradation in rat muscle by a glucocorticoid-dependent mechanism. J Clin Invest 1986; 77:614–621.
30. Maddox DA, Horn JF, Famiano FC, Gennari FJ. Load dependence of proximal tubular fluid and bicarbonate reabsorption in the remnant kidney of the Munich-Wistar rat. J Clin Invest 1986; 77:1639–1649.
31. Jarusiripipat C, Shapiro JI, Chan L, Schrier RW. Reduction of remnant nephron hypermetabolism by protein restriction. Am J Kidney Dis 1991; 18:367–374.
32. Schrier RW, Harris DCH, Chan L, Shapiro JI, Caramelo C. Tubular hypermetabolism as a factor in the progression of chronic renal failure. Am J Kidney Dis 1988; 12:243–249.
33. Nath KA, Croatt AJ, Hostetter TH. Oxygen consumption and oxidant stress in surviving nephrons. Am J Physiol 1990; 258:F1354–F1362.
34. Culpepper RM, Schoolwerth AC. Remnant kidney oxygen consumption: hypermetabolism or hyperbole? J Am Soc Nephrol 1992; 3:151–156.

5

Diabetic Nephropathy

Trond G. Jenssen   University Hospital of Tromsø, Tromsø, Norway

INTRODUCTION

Diabetes mellitus is one of the most frequent causes of renal failure in the Western world. In the United States, diabetes mellitus accounts for about 43% of all cases of end-stage renal disease (1). Some 30% of all patients with diabetes mellitus develop diabetic nephropathy, defined as proteinuria of more than 500 mg protein/24 h and/or a fall in glomerular filtration rate (GFR) (2).

Several pathogenic mechanisms are involved, including hemodynamic factors contributing to increased intraglomerular pressure, growth factors such as transforming growth factor beta (TGF-β) and platelet-derived growth factor (PDGF), and possibly also glycation products inducing altered cell function. The predisposition to develop diabetic nephropathy seems to be partly a genetic trait other than that of developing diabetes itself (3).

Before overt diabetic nephropathy develops, it is preceded by a period of intermediate urinary albumin excretion called microalbuminuria. Microalbuminuria is defined as an albumin excretion rate of 20–200 μg/min in timed urine samples or 2.5–25 mg/mmol

Table 1   Risk Factors for Development of Microalbuminuria: Results of the Tromsø Health Survey ($n = 4.385$)

Variable	Odds ratio	95% CI	$p <$
Hypertension	3.1	2.5–3.8	0.0001
Diabetes	3.1	2.0–4.8	0.0001
Smoking	2.5	2.0–3.1	0.0001
Male sex	1.8	1.4–2.2	0.0001
Age (by 10 years)	1.6	1.4–1.8	0.0001
Cardiovascular disease	1.3	1.0–1.7	0.020

Multiple logistic regression.

creatinine in spot urine (4). Up to 30–40% of microalbuminuric type I diabetics develop overt nephropathy over 8 years if untreated. In addition, microabuminuria predicts cardiovascular disease in both type I (5) and type II (6,7) diabetics.

In the Tromsø Health Survey, we relate the presence of microalbuminuria to risk factors and existing cardiovascular disease in the general population. Microalbuminuria is defined as an albumin/creatinine ratio of 2.5–25 mg/mmol in two of three sterile urine samples. Table 1 shows the independent risk factors for development of microalbuminuria in this study. As can be seen, hypertension, diabetes, and smoking are all strong and independent risk factors associated with the presence of microalbuminuria.

PRIMARY INTERVENTION

Primary intervention is directed toward preventing development of microalbuminuria in a diabetic person with presumably healthy kidneys. In the Tromsø Health Survey, there is a linear trend between the degree of albuminuria and HbA1C even in the nondiabetic range (data to be published). It is therefore no wonder that the only documented successful treatment in primary prevention of renal disease in diabetics is intensified blood-glucose control. Several studies published in the 1980s indicated this, but the final proof came with the Diabetes Control and Complications Trial (DCCT) published in 1993

(8). A total of 1441 patients with insulin-dependent diabetes mellitus (IDDM) were followed for a mean of 6.5 years. Half of them received intensified insulin treatment with an average HbA1C of 7%, the other half conventional morning and evening insulin with an average HbA1C of 9% (normal range <6.05%). Intensive therapy reduced the risk of developing microalbuminuria by 34%, and it also reduced the risk of developing retinopathy by 76% and neuropathy by 69% (8).

The DCCT gave convincing evidence that tight control of the blood sugar is essential to prevent microvascular complications, at least in type I diabetics. However, the trial has also initiated a debate over whether it is feasible for diabetics to maintain such control outside the framework of a clinical trial with all its resources. In this context, it is of interest to note that some centers report a decline in the accumulated incidence of diabetic nephropathy. In Linköping, Sweden, the accumulated incidence of diabetic nephropathy after 20 years of diabetic disease has declined from 30% in the 1961–65 cohort to 6% in the 1971–75 cohort (9). In the latter cohort, HbA1C has averaged 7.0–7.5% over the last 15 years (normal range <6.0%). Furthermore, improvement of blood-glucose control in IDDM patients not only prevents the development of microalbuminuria, it also slows the progression of morphological changes in the diabetic kidney (10).

SECONDARY INTERVENTION

Secondary intervention implies either preventing the microalbuminuric patient from progressing to overt proteinuria or delaying the progression of renal failure in patients with established nephropathy. The combined data from the DCCT indicate that tight glucose control is also essential in preventing progression of established microalbuminuria (8).

Microalbuminuria and ACE Inhibition

From a theoretical point of view, angiotensin-converting enzyme (ACE) inhibitors should have beneficial effects on the diabetic kidney, since they interfere with some of the mechanisms that seem to be essential in the pathogenesis of diabetic nephropathy. The agents reduce the systemic blood pressure; they lower the intraglomerular pressure through specific effects on the efferent glomerular sphincter; they seem to improve the molecular sieving coefficient in the glomerular basement membrane; and they have antigrowth effects. It is therefore not surprising that ACE inhibitors, compared to placebo, delay the progression of microalbuminuria in IDDM patients (11). However, it has been difficult to tell whether the beneficial effect on microalbuminuria can be ascribed solely to the antihypertensive effect of the ACE inhibitor or whether mechanisms more specific to the kidney are also operative.

Just recently, Viberti et al. (12) published the results on 2 years of treatment with captopril (50 mg × 2) in normotensive IDDM patients with microalbuminuria. All together, 235 patients participated in this placebo-controlled trial. The albumin excretion rate increased by 25% in the placebo group and fell by 31% in the captopril group. Twenty-two percent of the patients receiving placebo and only 7% of the patients receiving captopril developed overt proteinuria, defined as an albumin excretion rate $>200 \mu g/min$. The patients receiving captopril had slightly lower blood pressure throughout the trial compared to those receiving placebo, but even after correction for this discrepancy the risk of nephropathic progression was reduced by 63% in the captopril group. This indicates that mechanisms other than the systemic blood pressure are counteracted with ACE inhibition.

The most long-term follow-up data with ACE inhibition in normotensive microalbuminuric type I diabetics are those reported by Mathiesen et al. (13). Forty-four patients received either captopril or placebo for 8 years. Forty percent of the placebo group progressed to nephropathy, compared to only 10% in the captopril group. Several of the patients in the placebo group showed a decline in GFR once they developed nephropathy. This study indicates both that the effect of ACE inhibition on the kidney is long-lasting and that treatment of microalbuminuric type I diabetics with ACE inhibition, regardless of blood pressure, retards the development of renal failure.

Most studies dealing with normotensive microalbuminuric diabetic patients have addressed type I diabetics. However, a 5-year follow-up study from Israel (14) shows that the same effect can also be expected in normotensive type II diabetics.

Delaying the Progression of Diabetic Nephropathy

The purpose of intervention when renal function is already declining is to postpone the establishment of end-stage renal disease. During the course of the disease, the GFR falls by some 4–7 ml/min/yr. A reduced slope of the curve is desirable. Follow-up studies indicate a significant correlation between the rate of decline in renal function and the diastolic blood pressure once it exceeds 90 mm Hg (15).

In the middle of the 1980s, we received the first reports that efficient antihypertensive treatment delayed the progression of renal failure in IDDM patients with nephropathy (16,17). The rate of progression was retarded by some 50% once blood pressure was lowered below 140/90 mm Hg. Later reports showed that ACE inhibitors could have a renal protective effect in established diabetic nephropathy beyond the effect caused by blood-pressure reduction itself (18). The studies involved a limited number of patients, but a meta-analysis seemed to confirm the findings (19).

This question was addressed by the Collaborative Study Group, which followed 409 IDDM patients with established nephropathy (urinary protein excretion >500 mg/24 h). Half of the patients received captopril 25 mg × 3, half received placebo (20). Several patients in the placebo group received antihypertensive treatment, but not calcium channel blockers or ACE inhibitors, and the blood pressures of the two groups were fairly comparable. Captopril reduced the risk of doubling creatinine by 48%, and the risk of the combined endpoints death, dialysis, and transplantation by 50% (20). The effects persisted even after correction for differences in blood pressure.

Tight blood-pressure control is essential in diabetic patients with incipient or overt nephropathy, and ACE inhibitors are the drug of choice unless contraindicated by other causes.

Restriction of dietary protein has been advocated as a possible strategy to delay the development of end-stage renal failure. Smaller studies, dealing with 20–30 patients, have indicated that the GFR is better preserved in type I diabetics given a low-protein, low-phosphorus diet containing 0.6–0.7 g protein/kg body weight per day, as opposed to an ordinary diet of at least 1 g protein/kg body weight per day (21,22). The studies have followed the patients for up to 3 years. However, long-term studies beyond 3 years have not been performed in diabetics, and compliance represents a potential problem. The well-known Modification of Diet in Renal Disease (MDRD) trial, which followed more than 900 patients with nondiabetic renal failure for 3 years, did not show significant effects of protein restriction in this group of patients (23). However, diabetics with insulin requirements were not included in the study.

Another important point to consider before prescribing a complex treatment is whether the different regimens have additive effects. For instance, most studies on ACE inhibition have been performed on diabetics with rather poor metabolic control. Theoretically, ACE inhibition and improved blood-glucose control could work through similar mechanisms, such as reducing hyperfiltration. The same could be said about protein restriction in the diet. Since we do not know the exact benefit of adding up the regimens, we should stick to those that are best documented.

Improved blood-glucose control prevents the development of microalbuminuria. ACE inhibition should be started in both type I and type II diabetics once microalbuminuria is confirmed, even when blood pressure is within the normal range.

In a recent paper from Manto et al. (24), 14 IDDM patients with nephropathy, followed for 36 months, received a combined therapy of improved glucose control (HbA1C 6.5%), ACE inhibition (blood pressure averaging 120/75 mm Hg), and low-protein diet (0.8 g/kg/day). During the course of the study, GFR increased and urinary albumin excretion rate decreased (24). These are promising results, but they are rather difficult to interpret because the study did not involve a control group.

PROSPECTS FOR THE FUTURE

Extensive data from animal studies show that a mediating mechanism of microvascular complications in diabetes can be the nonenzymatic binding of excess glucose to body proteins, lipids, and nucleic acids. These compounds are called advanced glycation end-products (AGE).

Their physiology and possible role in disease are extensively reviewed elsewhere (25). The AGE modification is irreversible and highly reactive, inducing, for example, cross-link formation between polypeptides of collagen, oxidation of lipids, and inactivation of nitrous oxide. Treatment of diabetic animals with either AGE antibodies or aminoguanidine, an inhibitor of AGE formation and an inhibitor of nitrous oxide synthase, delays or prevents the development of nephropathy in animals (26,27). These are promising results, and aminoguanidine is now the subject of ongoing studies in humans.

The lipid profile in diabetic subjects is characterized by low HDL cholesterol and elevated VLDL cholesterol and triglycerides. Numerous studies in nondiabetics have found a close correlation between lipid abnormalities and the development of kidney disease. Animal studies show that hyperlipidemia induces glomerular damage similar to cholesterol-induced changes in large arteries, and lipid-lowering treatment prevents glomerulosclerosis from developing in hyperlipidemic animals (for a review, see Ref. 28). We do not yet have intervention data to tell us whether a similar approach will have beneficial effects in diabetic humans. However, we do know that lipid-lowering treatment with HMG-CoA-reductase inhibitors in diabetics with coronary artery disease reduces their risk of death over 5.5 years from 25 to 14%, compared to 11 and 8%, respectively, in nondiabetics with coronary artery disease (29). Therefore, diabetic patients with coronary artery disease and hyperlipidemia should receive lipid-lowering treatment, to save their lives if not their kidneys.

In conclusion, several pathogenic mechanisms including hemodynamic changes, glycation, and growth factors are operative in diabetic nephropathy. Primary prevention of microalbuminuria involves tight glucose control, whereas ACE inhibition should be started once microalbuminuria or overt proteinuria are established. We are still short of data on the combined effects of tight glucose control, antihypertensive treatment, and dietary protein restriction.

REFERENCES

1. Perneger TV, Brancati FL, Whelton PK, Klag MJ. End-stage renal disease attributable to diabetes mellitus. Ann Intern Med 1994; 121:912–918.

2. Andersen AR, Christiansen JS, Andersen JK, Kreiner S, Deckert T. Diabetic nephropathy in type I (insulin dependent) diabetes: an epidemiological study. Diabetologia 1983; 25:496–501.

3. Seaquist ER, Goetz FC, Rich S, Barbosa J. Familial clustering of diabetic kidney disease: evidence for genetic susceptibility to diabetic nephropathy. N Engl J Med 1989; 320:1161–1165.

4. Mogensen CE, Keane WF, Bennett PH, Jerums G, Parving H-H, Passa P, Steffes MW, Striker GE, Viberti GC. Prevention of diabetic renal disease with special reference to microalbuminuria. Lancet 1995; 346: 1080–1084.

5. Messent JW, et al. Prognostic significance of microalbuminuria in insulin-dependent diabetes mellitus: a twenty-three year follow up study. Kidney Int 1992; 41:836–839.

6. Jarrett RJ, Viberti GC, Argyropoulos A, Hill RD, Mahmud U, Murrells TJ. Microalbuminuria predicts mortality in non-insulin-dependent diabetes. Diabetic Med 1984; 1:17–19.

7. Mogensen CE. Microalbuminuria predicts clinical proteinuria and early mortality in maturity-onset diabetes. N Engl J Med 1984; 310: 356–360.

8. The Diabetes Control and Complications Trial Research Group. The effect of intensive treatment of diabetes on the development and progression of long-term complications in insulin-dependent mellitus. N Engl J Med 1993; 329:977–986.

9. Bojestig M, Arnqvist HJ, Hermansson G, Karlberg BE, Ludvigsson J. Declining incidence of nephropathy in insulin-dependent diabetes mellitus. N Engl J Med 1994; 330:15–18.

10. Bangstad H-J, Østerby R, Dahl-Jørgensen K, Berg KJ, Hartmann A, Hanssen KF. Improvement of blood glucose control in IDDM patients retards the progression of morphological changes in early diabetic nephropathy. Diabetologia 1994; 37:483–490.

11. Marre M, Chatellier G, Leblanc H, Guyene TT, Menard J, Passa P. Prevention of diabetic nephropathy with enalapril in normotensive diabetics with microalbuminuria. Br Med J 1988; 297:1092–1095.

12. Viberti GC, Laffel L, Gans DJ. Secondary prevention of diabetic nephropathy by captopril in patients with insulin-dependent diabetes mellitus (IDDM) and microalbuminuria. J Am Soc Nephrol 1994; 5:385.

13. Mathiesen ER, Hommel E, Smith U, Parving H-H. Efficacy of captopril in normotensive diabetic patients with microalbuminuria—8 years follow up. Diabetologia 1995; 38(suppl 1):A46.

14. Ravid M, Savin H, Jutrin I, Bental T, Katz B, Lishner M. Long-term stabilizing effect of angiotensin-converting enzyme inhibition on plas-

ma creatinine and on proteinuria in normotensive type II diabetic patients. Ann Intern Med 1993; 118:577–581.

15. Rossing P, Hommel E, Smidt UM, Parving H-H. Impact of arterial blood pressure and albuminuria on the progression of diabetic nephropathy in IDDM patients. Diabetes 1993; 42:715–719.

16. Mogensen CE. Long-term antihypertensive treatment inhibiting progression of diabetic nephropathy. Br Med J 1982; 285:685–688.

17. Parving H-H, Andersen AR, Smidt UM, Hommel E, Mathiesen ER, Svendsen PA. Effect of antihypertensive treatment on kidney function in diabetic nephropathy. Br Med J 1987; 294:1443–1447.

18. Bjørck S, Mulec H, Johnsen SA, Nyberg G, Aurell M. Contrasting effects of enalapril and metoprolol on proteinuria in diabetic nephropathy. Br Med J 1990; 300:904–907.

19. Kasiske BL, Kalil RSN, Ma JZ, Liao M, Keane WF. Effect of antihypertensive therapy on the kidney in patients with diabetes: a meta-regression analysis. Ann Intern Med 1993; 118:129–138.

20. Lewis EJ, Hunsicker LG, Bain RP, Rohde RD. The effect of angiotensin-converting-enzyme inhibition on diabetic nephropathy. N Engl J Med 1993; 329:1456–1462.

21. Walker JD, Bending JJ, Dodds RA, Mattock MB, Murrells TJ, Keen H, Viberti GC. Restriction of dietary protein and progression of renal failure in diabetic nephropathy. Lancet 1989; ii:1411–1415.

22. Zeller K, Whittaker E, Sullivan L, Raskin P, Jacobson HR. Effect of restricting dietary protein on the progression of renal failure in patients with insulin-dependent diabetes mellitus. N Engl J Med 1991; 324: 78–84.

23. Klahr S, Levey AS, Beck GJ, Caggiula AW, Hunsicker L, Kusek JW, Striker G. The effects of dietary protein restriction and blood-pressure control on the progression of chronic renal disease. N Engl J Med 1994; 330:877–884.

24. Manto A, Cotroneo P, Marra G, Magnani P, Tilli P, Greco AV, Ghirlanda G. Effect of intensive treatment on diabetic nephropathy in patients with type I diabetes. Kidney Int 1995; 47:231–235.

25. Vlassara H, Bucala R, Striker L. Pathogenic effects of advanced glycosylation: biochemical, biologic, and clinical implications for diabetes and aging. Lab Invest 1994; 70:138–151.

26. Cohen MP, Hud E, Wu V-Y. Amelioration of diabetic nephropathy by treatment with monoclonal antibodies against glycated albumin. Kidney Int 1994; 45:1673–1679.

27. Soulis-Liparota T, Cooper M, Papazoglou D, Clarke B, Jerums G. Retardation by aminoguanidine of development of albuminuria, mesan-

gial expansion, and tissue fluorescence in streptozocin-induced diabetic rat. Diabetes 1991; 40:1328–1334.
28. Keane WF, Kasiske BL, O'Donnell MP, Kim Y. The role of altered
    lipid metabolism in the progression of renal disease: experimental evi-
    dence. Am J Kidney Dis 1991; 17(suppl 1):38–42.
29. Pyörälä K, Pedersen TR, Kjekshus J. The effect of cholesterol lowering
    with simvastatin on coronary events in diabetic patients with coronary
    heart disease. Diabetes 1995; 44(suppl 1):35A.

6

Etiology and Pathophysiology of Left Ventricular Hypertrophy

Franz H. Messerli and Leszek Michalewicz   Ochsner Clinic and Alton Ochsner Medical Foundation, New Orleans, Louisiana

INTRODUCTION

Left ventricular hypertrophy (LVH) is defined as an increase in the muscle mass of the left ventricle. Hypertension, obesity, advanced age, valvular heart diseases, renal disease, and other pathological disorders can lead to LVH (Figure 1) (1,2). Conceivably, an increased left ventricular mass could represent a "final common pathway" (3) epitomizing the adverse effects of a variety of influences on the cardiovascular system.

Initially, in hypertension or other cardiovascular disorders, LVH may be benign and compensatory. According to Laplace's law, the degree of left ventricular wall stress is directly proportional to the intracavitary pressure and the radius of the chamber and is inversely proportional to wall thickness, so an increase in wall thickness decreases ventricular wall stress (4–9). Unfortunately, no reliable symptoms or signs allow one to distinguish between compensatory and pathological LVH. Clearly, however, LVH is not simply a compensatory

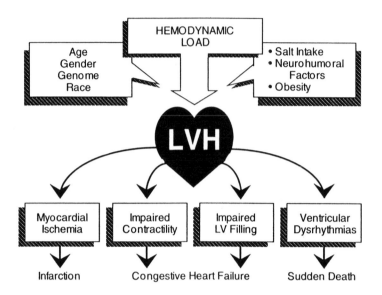

Figure 1   Determinants and cardiac sequelae of LVH. (From Ref. 2.)

mechanism. The increase in myocardial mass lowers coronary reserve and enhances cardiac oxygen requirements. The Framingham Heart Study (8,9) has documented that the risk of acute myocardial infarction, congestive heart failure, sudden death, and other cardiovascular events increases six- to eightfold with the occurrence of LVH. LVH has proven to be an extremely powerful predictor of poor prognosis regardless of whether it occurs in hypertensive patients or in the general population (10–13).

MORPHOLOGICAL PATTERNS OF LVH

The classic form of LVH, concentric hypertrophy, is defined as a thickening of the septum and the posterior wall of the left ventricle at the expense of chamber volume, which is the typical ventricular adaptation to an increase in afterload that occurs after long-standing hypertension (14–17). It occurs by replication of sarcomeres and increase of cell width without increasing the number of myocytes

(18– 20) and is associated as well with increase and remodeling of extracellular collagen (21–23) and with growth of fibroblasts (24–27). In the cell level, changes in expression of proto-oncogenes and other genes that regulate cell growth and differentiation take place (28–31). With increasing duration and severity of hypertension, relative wall thickness (wall thickness divided by left ventricular dimension) increases as well. The significance of concentric remodeling of the left ventricle (increased relative wall thickness with normal left ventricular mass) is still controversial; data from a Framingham cohort, however, suggest that increased cardiovascular risk is associated with this type of altered ventricular geometry (32).

Eccentric LVH, defined as thickening of the chamber wall with concomitant chamber dilatation, occurs in the late phase of hypertensive heart disease and is a precursor of congestive heart failure. Eccentric LVH is also seen with other pathological conditions characterized by fluid volume overload, such as obesity, mitral and aortic regurgitation, and renal insufficiency (33–35). According to Laplace's law, chamber dilatation increases ventricular wall stress and therefore leads to an increase in muscle mass (6) (Figure 2).

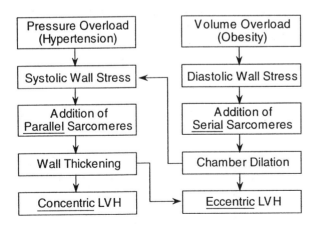

Figure 2 Pathogenesis of left ventricular hypertrophy in obesity and hypertension. (From Ref. 36.)

Table 1   Effects of Pathological LVH vs. Physiological LVH on Ventricular
Ectopy, Coronary Reserve, Ventricular Filling, and Myocardial Fibrosis

	Pathological LVH	Physiological LVH
Ventricular ectopy	Increased	None
Coronary reserve	Diminished	Normal or increased
Ventricular filling	Impaired	Normal or increased
Myocardial fibrosis	Common	Absent

Source: Modified from Ref. 43.

Increased muscle mass of the left ventricle can also be found in athletes as a structural adaptation to regular exercise (37–41). An eccentric type of LVH with increased cardiac contractile reserve is observed in athletes undergoing dynamic exercise, such as runners. With dynamic exercise, little or no wall thickening occurs, depending on the number of muscles used. In contrast, isometric exercise (e.g., weightlifting) results in an increase in wall thickness with a normal cavity size (42) and often results in a morphological pattern similar to asymmetrical septal hypertrophy. Although the physiological LVH that occurs with dynamic exercise can clearly be differentiated from the pathological hypertrophy that occurs in essential hypertension (Table 1) (43), the clinical and prognostic significance of the changes in left ventricular geometry associated with isometric exercise is still controversial (44).

PREVALENCE AND DIAGNOSIS OF LVH

The prevalence of LVH is far greater than is generally appreciated. Early data from the Framingham Heart Study (45) suggested that one in 10 persons will have LVH at the ages of 65 to 69, as determined by electrocardiography. Because electrocardiography lacks specificity and sensitivity (46,47), echocardiography has become the diagnostic procedure of choice over the last decade, confirming and expanding our knowledge about LVH (48–50). Data derived by echocardiography from the Framingham cohort (51) demonstrated a prevalence of LVH of 16% for men and 19% for women, increasing after the age of 70 to 33% for men and 49% for women. Echocardiographic data from Hammond et al. (52) have shown an overall LVH prevalence of 20% for patients with mild hypertension. With more severe essential hypertension, the prevalence may reach 50% (53, 54).

Although elevated arterial pressure is undoubtedly the main factor in the development of LVH, the actual correlation between left ventricular mass and arterial pressure is surprisingly poor, particularly for casual blood pressures (55). When intra-arterial systolic blood pressure was correlated with LVH in our laboratory, a somewhat better correlation of 0.42 was found (56). The best correlations, however, have been found between certain indices of ambulatory blood pressure monitoring and LVH. Several studies have shown that blood pressure during the day or during daytime work is more closely correlated with LVH than blood pressure during sleep or at rest (57–61), with the correlation generally being less close for diastolic than for systolic pressures. Other indices derived from ambulatory blood-pressure monitoring and currently being investigated as tools in the prediction of LVH include the blood-pressure load (the percentage of blood-pressure readings about the certain limit, usually 140 mm Hg systolic and 90 mm Hg diastolic) (62) and the tension time index (the product of systolic blood pressure and ejection time determined in relation to the heart rate) (63).

DETERMINANTS OF LVH

The poor correlation between arterial pressure and left ventricular mass indicates that the increased hemodynamic burden on the heart is not the sole determinant of left ventricular structure. Indeed, other factors have been suggested that may independently influence the development of LVH (64).

Age

Many studies have indicated that left ventricular wall thickness and left ventricular mass increase with age (65–67). Although this increase was thought to be a sign of an intrinsic myocardial aging process, a detailed analysis of the relationship of age to left ventricular mass in a healthy subset of the Framingham Study population suggests that the relationship is a function of other extramyocardial events, such as elevated blood pressure, obesity, valvular disease, and occult coronary artery disease, that tend to increase with age (68,69). A recent multicenter trial (70) confirmed these findings and found no association of age with wall thickness or left ventricular mass after adjustment for blood pressure and body mass index.

Gender

It is now well established that women have a smaller left ventricular mass than men for any given level of arterial pressure (71,72), even when correlated for body-surface area, which indicates that sex hormones may influence myocardial adaptation to a given hemodynamic load. Endogenous androgens appear to exert a trophic effect on the cardiac muscle, as demonstrated by animal studies (73), and estrogen activity may exert a preventive or even protective effect with regard to the development of LVH. In addition, a recent study suggested that there might be sex-specific differences in the development of LVH, even in patients without hypertension (74–76). Increased sympathetic nervous system activity was found to be the only significant determinant in normotensive men, whereas in women increased adiposity seemed to be the predominant factor associated with LVH.

Race

Although the reasons are still unclear, black patients are known to have a higher prevalence of hypertension than white patients (77), as well as more frequent hypertensive complications such as sudden death, congestive heart failure, stroke, and renal failure. Studies (78–80) have documented that for any level of blood pressure, black patients have more severe hypertensive target organ damage than white patients. We previously demonstrated that the posterior wall was thicker, and most important, left ventricular mass was greater in black patients than in white patients with similar blood pressure levels (81).

Obesity

An increase in body mass resulting from increased adipose tissue requires a higher cardiac output and an expanded intravascular volume to meet the higher metabolic demands. Therefore, cardiac adaptation to obesity results in LVH of the eccentric type (i.e., an increase in myocardial mass combined with chamber dilatation) (34, 82–85). We previously demonstrated that, compared with lean subjects, obese subjects with the same arterial pressure have distinctly elevated left ventricular diameters and wall thickness as well as increased left ventricular mass (i.e., eccentric LVH) (86). Data from the Framingham cohort (45) demonstrated a nine- to tenfold increase in prevalence of LVH, depending on the grade of obesity. In addition, a recent study (87) suggested that indices of central obesity, such as waist circumference and the waist-to-hip ratio, are important and independent predictors of LVH.

Salt Intake

The INTERSALT study (88) demonstrated that daily urinary sodium excretion and blood pressure are related. Animal studies (89) have demonstrated that high sodium intake results in a blood-pressure-independent increase in heart weight, and that restriction of sodium reverses the increase in relative heart weight but does not reverse the increase in blood pressure.

We identified salt intake as a strong determinant of LVH (90). With sodium excretion as a measure of dietary salt intake, a close correlation was found between sodium excretion and diastolic diameter of the left chamber and, more important, left ventricular mass. These observations suggest that dietary salt intake is a blood-pressure-independent determinant of the degree of myocardial hypertrophy. These findings have subsequently been confirmed by a number of other investigators (70,91–93) and expanded to different subsets of the population, such as hypertensive children and adolescents (94,95), hypertensive elderly (96), and normotensive persons (97–99).

Alcohol Intake

Although recent data derived from the INTERSALT study indicate a significant relationship between alcohol intake and hypertension (100), the association of alcohol with LVH is less clear. Although heavy drinking has been found to have a small but significant positive association with left ventricular mass, as reported by Framingham cohort (101), other investigators could not find such a relationship (70,102).

Job Strain

Job strain defined as high psychological demands and low decision latitude on the job was found to be significantly related to hypertension and LVH (57,58,103).

Neurohumoral Factors

Various neurohumoral influences, particularly the renin-angiotensin and adrenergic systems, insulin, growth factors, and genetic factors may play important roles in the pathogenesis of LVH (104–113). The effect of angiotensin-converting enzyme inhibitors (ACEI) causing regression of LVH and preventing remodeling after myocardial infarction confirms the importance of the renin angiotensin system (114–117). A very important issue is the existence of the tissue angiotensin system (118). Each component of the renin angiotensin system (except, perhaps renin) is also synthesized locally in the ventricle (119,120). The ability of doses of ACE inhibitors that do not lower blood pressure to produce regression in LVH supports the hypothesis that the local cardiac angiotensin system is significant in determining heart structure and function (114,121–124). Elevated levels of aldosterone are associated with myocardial fibrosis (15). The effects of growth factors may be transmitted by the $alpha_1$-adrenergic receptor to activate intracellular transducing proteins and ribonucleic acid (RNA) transcription factors (125,126). Growth factors are multifunctional and can either inhibit or stimulate growth of cells (127).

SPECIFIC CONSIDERATIONS IN RENAL FAILURE

The functions of the renal and cardiovascular systems are very closely related. A variety of renal diseases commonly attack the cardiovascular condition, and, conversely, cardiovascular complications may also occur in patients with renal disease who had no preexisting cardiovascular problems; cardiac and vascular lesions are the most frequent complications observed in those patients (23,128–134). Various renal mechanisms are involved in pathogenesis of essential hypertension (135), and chronic renal disease is the most common cause of secondary hypertension. Both hypertension and diabetes mellitus accelerate atherosclerosis and are leading causes of end-stage renal disease (136,137).

In patients with renal insufficiency, pressure overload may occur due to increased stiffness and decreased distensibility of aorta and other arteries (138), abnormalities in the renin-angiotensin system (139,140), and absence of vasodepressors of renal origin (141). As discussed before, a pressure overload will result in concentric remodeling of the left ventricle.

Other pathophysiological factors related to renal insufficiency cause chronic volume and flow overload. Among them are sodium and water retention (142), A-V shunts (143,144), and anemia. Chronic anemia is associated with an increase in heart rate, stroke volume, and cardiac output. The systemic resistances are low because of a decrease in blood viscosity and vasodilatation (145–147). These factors will lead to eccentric remodeling. Thus, the heart in renal failure is characterized by both concentric and eccentric hypertrophy.

Additional factors that influence cardiac function and structured in uremic patients are secondary hyperparathyroidism (148–150) and proliferation of fibrous tissue (151).

CARDIAC SEQUELAE OF LVH

Ventricular Filling

Impaired left ventricular filling has been documented as an early finding in hypertensive heart disease (152). Initially, decreased filling may be due to impaired relaxation; as a consequence, the rapid in-flow of blood into the left ventricle in early diastole is diminished and shifted toward later diastole. With progressive LVH, however, late diastolic compliance also diminishes. As demonstrated by Sax et al. (153), the ventricle becomes progressively stiffer and therefore re-quires a higher filling pressure to maintain a similar ejection fraction. Impaired diastolic filling usually is well compensated for under rest-ing conditions but may lead to symptoms and signs of congestive heart failure during exercise.

Of note, as left ventricular mass increases secondary to aerobic exercise, left ventricular filling remains unchanged or even improves (154). Thus, in hypertensive patients and endurance-trained athletes, left ventricular mass may be the same, but left ventricular filling is likely to be different. Impaired left ventricular filling is the hallmark that separates physiological from pathological hypertrophy.

Myocardial Contractility and Congestive Heart Failure

Congestive heart failure is known to be a common complication of untreated longstanding hypertension. Data from the Framingham Heart Study (155) have shown that more than 80% of patients with manifest congestive heart failure had elevated blood-pressure levels. Thus, as hypertensive cardiovascular disease progresses, the hyper-trophied heart is no longer able to compensate for an ever-increasing afterload. The left heart chamber becomes dilated, and a decrease in ejection fraction and cardiac output can be observed. The increased activity of the sympathetic nervous system and the renin-angiotensin system serves to stabilize arterial pressure. Vasoconstriction that leads to myocardial ischemia further impairs pump function and ac-celerates the fall in contractility. Congestive heart failure ensues.

Sax et al. (153) demonstrated that an increase in chamber stiff-ness can lead to clinically manifested heart failure in the presence of normal systolic function. Similarly, Topol et al. (152) documented supernormal systolic function in a group of elderly hypertensive pa-tients with heart failure. In these studies, however, left ventricular function was usually assessed by endocardial fractional fiber shortening rather than by the physiologically more appropriate midwall fiber shortening. By taking into account the relative movement of the midwall toward the epicardium in systole, de Simone et al. (156, 157) recently demonstrated that hypertensive patients with either concentric remodeling or concentric hypertrophy show decreased ventricular function according to midwall fiber shortening. Pathologically decompensation due to volume or pressure overload is associated with degeneration and lysis of myofibrils (21,158,159).

Thus, whether systolic or diastolic dysfunction is more important or more prevalent in the pathogenesis of congestive heart failure in patients with LVH and longstanding hypertension remains to be documented.

Myocardial Ischemia

Myocardial ischemia has been shown to be common among hypertensive patients with LVH. A variety of pathogenetic mechanisms may be responsible. First, hypertension has been directly implicated in the pathogenesis of coronary atherosclerosis, which further impedes myocardial oxygen supply. Second, in hypertensive patients who have not yet developed LVH, exaggerated reactivity of the cardiac arterioles has been documented, leading to the clinical picture of "microvascular angina." Third, both an increase in arterial pressure, resulting from increased hemodynamic burden of the heart, and an increase in left ventricular mass require more oxygen for tissue perfusion. Lastly, the growth of capillary beds in the hypertrophying myocardium does not keep pace with the increasing left ventricular mass (160–163). Strauer (164,165) showed that coronary reserve (the difference between the basal and maximal coronary blood flow during maximal coronary vasodilatation) decreased in patients with LVH, even when their coronary arteries were patent on coronary angiograms. Similarly, Tomanek et al. (166) and Marcus et al. (167) demonstrated that certain types of cardiac hypertrophy are associated with major abnormalities in coronary reserve. Pichard et al. (168) found a relationship between the decrease in coronary reserve and the degree of LVH. The findings of Strauer (169) indicated that the impairment of coronary reserve is not due to LVH per se but rather to structural changes in coronary arteries. Silent myocardial ischemia has been shown to be independent of left ventricular mass in hypertensive patients and to be influenced predominantly by wall stress (170).

Ventricular Ectopy

As early as 1984, we reported that hypertensive patients with LVH have a significantly greater prevalence of premature ventricular contractions and complex ventricular arrhythmias than do patients without LVH or normotensive patients (171), a finding that was later expanded to obese patients with eccentric LVH (172) and confirmed in large population-based studies (51,173). Although it is still controversial whether these findings could explain at least in part the higher incidence of sudden cardiac death in these patients, a study from the Framingham cohort (174,175) indicated recently that in patients with LVH, the presence of asymptomatic ventricular arrhythmias was indeed associated with a nearly twofold increase in mortality.

The mechanism by which LVH leads to increased arrhythmogenicity and ultimately to increased mortality remains unknown. A variety of factors associated with LVH are currently being considered as possible mechanisms, such as reduced coronary flow reserve, silent myocardial ischemia, abnormal electrophysiological properties of hypertrophied myocytes, or conduction disturbances because of increased fibrous tissue or altered collagen content (167,176–181).

CONCLUSIONS

LVH has been identified as a significant independent risk factor and a harbinger of sudden death, myocardial infarction, congestive heart failure, and other events leading to cardiovascular morbidity and mortality. Whether a reduction of LVH will ultimately improve this ominous prognosis remains unclear; a recent study from the Framingham cohort, however, suggests that regression of electrocardiographic features of LVH confers an improvement in risk of cardiovascular diseases; worsening of these features imposes increased risk. In general, this holds true for both voltage criteria of LVH and repolarization abnormalities. Other studies indicate that the reduction of LVH diminishes ventricular arrhythmias (172), improves ventricular filling, and preserves or even improves left ventricular function. Hopefully, prospective epidemiological studies will document the benefits of such a targeted therapeutic approach (182).

REFERENCES

1. Messerli FH, Ketelhut R. Left ventricular hypertrophy: an independent risk factor. J Cardiovasc Pharmacol 1991; 17(suppl 4):S59–S67.
2. Messerli FH, Soria F. Hypertension, left ventricular hypertrophy, ventricular ectopy, and sudden death. Am J Med 1992; 93(suppl 2A):21–26S.
3. Devereux RB. Does increased blood pressure cause left ventricular hypertrophy or vice-versa? [editorial]. Ann Intern Med 1990; 112:157–159.
4. Lavie CJ, Ventura HO, Messerli FH. Regression of increased left ventricular mass by antihypertensives. Drugs 1991; 42:945–961.
5. Lavie CJ, Ventura HO, Messerli FH. Left ventricular hypertrophy: its relationship to obesity and hypertension. Postgrad Med 1992; 91:131–143.
6. Lavie CJ, Messerli FH. Cardiovascular adaptation to obesity and hypertension. Chest 1986; 90:275–279.
7. Aurigemma GP, Silver KH, Priest MA, Gaasch WH. Geometric changes allow normal ejection fraction despite depressed myocardial shortening in hypertensive left ventricular hypertrophy. J Am Coll Cardiol 1995; 26(1):195–202.
8. Kannel WB. Prevalence and natural history of electrocardiographic left ventricular hypertrophy. Am J Med 1983; 75(suppl 3a):4–11.
9. Krumholz HM, Larson M, Levy D. Prognosis of left ventricular geometric patterns in the Framingham Heart Study. J Am Coll Cardiol 1995; 25:879–884.
10. Levy D, Garrison RJ, Savage DD, et al. Left ventricular mass an incidence of coronary heart disease in an elderly cohort: the Framingham Heart Study. Ann Intern Med 1989; 110:101–107.
11. Bikkina M, Levy D, Evans JC, et al. Left ventricular mass and risk of stroke in an elderly cohort: the Framingham Heart Study. JAMA 1994; 272:33–36.

12. Gardin JM, Wagenknecht LE, Anton-Culver H, Flack J, et al. Relationship of cardiovascular risk factors to echocardiographic left ventricular mass in healthy young black and white adult men and women—the CARDIA study: Coronary Artery Risk Development in Young Adults. Circulation 1995; 92:380–387.

13. Shigematsu Y, Hamada M, Mukai M, Matsuoka H, et al. Clinical evidence for an association between left ventricular geometric adaptation and extracardiac target organ damage in essential hypertension. J Hypertens 1995; 13:155–160.

14. Messerli FH. Clinical determinants and manifestations of left ventricular hypertrophy. In: Messerli FH, ed. The Heart and Hypertension. New York: Yorke Medical Books, 1987:219.

15. Tarazi RC. The heart in hypertension [editorial]. N Engl J Med 1985; 312:308–309.

16. Tarazi RC, Frohlich ED. Is reversal of cardiac hypertrophy a desirable goal of antihypertensive therapy? Circulation 1987; 75:I-113–I-117.

17. Verdecchia P, Schillaci G, Borgioni C, Ciucci A, et al. Gender, day–night blood pressure changes, and left ventricular mass in essential hypertension: dippers and peakers. Am J Hypertens 1995; 8:193–196.

18. Anversa P, Ricci R, Olivetti G. Quantitative structural analysis of the myocardium during physiologic growth and induced cardiac hypertrophy: a review. J Am Coll Cardiol 1986; 7:1140–1149.

19. Francalanci P, Gallo P, Bernucci P, Silver MD, d'Amati G. The pattern of desmin filaments in myocardial disarray. Hum Pathol 1995; 26:262–266.

20. Yamamoto S, James TN, Sawada K, Okabe M, Kawamura K. Generation of new intercellular junctions between cardiocytes: a possible mechanism compensating for mechanical overload in the hypertrophied human adult myocardium. Circ Res 1996; 78:362–370.

21. Jalil JE, Doering CW, Janicki JS, Pick R, Schroff SG, Weber KT. Fibrillar collagen and myocardial stiffness in the intact hypertrophied rat left ventricle. Circ Res 1989; 64:1041–1050.

22. Abrahams C, Janicki JS, Weber KT. Myocardial hypertrophy in Macaca fascicularis: structural remodeling of the collagen matrix. Lab Invest 1987; 56:676–683.

23. Weber KT, Janicki JS, Shroff SG, Pick R, Chen RM, Bashey RI. Collagen remodeling of the pressure-overloaded, hypertrophied nonhuman primate myocardium. Circ Res 1988; 62:757–765.

24. Weber KT, Brill CG. Pathological hypertrophy and cardiac interstitium: fibrosis and renin-angiotensin-aldosterone system. Circulation 1991; 83:1849–1865.

25. Weber KT, Janicki JS, Pick R, Capasso J, Anversa P. Myocardial fibrosis and pathologic hypertrophy in the rat with renovascular hypertension. Am J Cardiol 1990; 65(suppl):1G–7G.
26. Brilla CG, Maisch B, Zhou G, Weber KT. Hormonal regulation of cardiac fibroblast function. Eur Heart J 1995; 16(suppl C):45–50.
27. Diez J, Laviades C, Monreal I, Gil MJ, et al. Toward the biochemical assessment of myocardial fibrosis in hypertensive patients. Am J Cardiol 1995; 76:14D–17D.
28. Varmus HE. The molecular genetics of cellular oncogenes. Annu Rev Genet 1984; 18:553–612.
29. Katan M, Parker PJ. Oncogenes and cell control. Nature 1988; 332: 203.
30. Varmus HE. Oncogenes and transcriptional control. Science 1987; 238: 1337–1339.
31. Charlemagne D, Swynghedauw B. Myocardial phenotypic changes in Na+, K+ ATPase in left ventricular hypertrophy: pharmacological consequences. Eur Heart J 1995; 16:20–23.
32. Koren MJ, Devereux RB, Casale PN, et al. Relation of left ventricular mass and geometry to morbidity and mortality in uncomplicated essential hypertension. Ann Intern Med 1991; 114:345–352.
33. de Simone G, Di Lorenzo L, Moccia D, et al. Hemodynamic hypertrophied left ventricular patterns in systemic hypertension. Am J Cardiol 1987; 60:1317–1321.
34. Messerli FH, Sundgaard-Riise K, Reisin ED, et al. Dimorphic cardiac adaptation to obesity and arterial hypertension. Ann Intern Med 1983; 99:757–761.
35. Cohen MV, Diaz P, Scheuer J. Echocardiographic assessment of left ventricular function in patients with chronic uremia. Clin Nephrol 1979; 12:156–162.
36. Messerli FH, Weidmann P, Reisin E, Aepfelbacher FC. Pathogenesis of left ventricular hypertrophy in obesity and hypertension. In: Zanchetti A, ed. Handbook of Hypertension—Pathophysiology and Hypertension. Amsterdam: Elsevier Science Publishing, 1996, in press.
37. Colan SD. Mechanics of left ventricular systolic and diastolic function in physiologic hypertrophy of the athlete heart [review]. Cardiol Clin 1992; 10:227–240.
38. Iglesias Cubero G, Rodriguez Reguero JJ, Terrados N, Gonzalez V, et al. Aldosterone levels and cardiac hypertrophy in professional cyclists. Int J Sports 1995; 16:475–477.

39. George KP, Wolfe LA, Burggraf GW, Norman R. Electrocardiographic and echocardiographic characteristics of female athletes. Med Sci Sports Exerc 1995; 27:1362–1370.
40. Rodriguez Reguero JJ, Iglesias Cubero G, Lopez de la Iglesia J, Terrados N, et al. Prevalence and upper limit of cardiac hypertrophy in professional cyclists. Eur J Appl Physiol 1995; 70:375–378.
41. Kokkinos PF, Narayan P, Colleran JA, Pittaras A, et al. Effects of regular exercise on blood pressure and left ventricular hypertrophy in African-American men with severe hypertension. N Engl J Med 1995; 333:1462–1467.
42. Colan SD, Sanders SP, Borow KM. Physiologic hypertrophy: effects on left ventricular systolic mechanics in athletes. J Am Coll Cardiol 1987; 9:776–783.
43. Messerli FH, Ketelhut R. Left ventricular hypertrophy: how important a risk factor? Cardiovasc Risk Factors 1990; 1:8–13.
44. Maron BJ, Pelliccia A, Spirito P. Cardiac disease in young trained athletes: insights into methods for distinguishing athlete's heart from structural heart disease, with particular emphasis on hypertrophic cardiomyopathy. Circulation 1995; 91:1596–1601.
45. Kannel WB, Gordon T, Offutt D. Left ventricular hypertrophy by electrocardiogram: prevalence, incidence, and mortality in the Framingham Study. Ann Intern Med 1969; 71:89–105.
46. Levy D, Salomon M, D'Agostino RB, Belanger M, Kannel BW. Prognostic implications of baseline electrocardiographic features and their serial change in subjects with electrocardiographic left ventricular hypertrophy. Circulation 1994; 90:1786–1793.
47. Okin PM, Roman MJ, Devereux RB, Kligfield P. Electrocardiographic identification of left ventricular hypertrophy: test performance in relation to definition of hypertrophy and presence of obesity. J Am Coll Cardiol 1996; 27:124–131.
48. Schiller NB. Two-dimensional echocardiography is preferable for measuring left ventricular mass: all that glitters is not a reference standard. Am J Card Imaging 1995; 9:203–205.
49. Crow RS, Prineas RJ, Rautaharju P, Hannan P, Liebson PR. Relation between electrocardiography and echocardiography for left ventricular mass in mild systemic hypertension (results from Treatment of Mild Hypertension Study). Am J Cardiol 1995; 75:1233–1238.
50. Abergel E, Tase M, Bohlender J, Menard J, Chatellier G. Which definition for echocardiographic left ventricular hypertrophy? Am J Cardiol 1995; 75:498–502.

51. Levy D, Anderson KM, Savage DD, et al. Echocardiographically detected left ventricular hypertrophy: prevalence and risk factors—the Framingham Heart Study. Ann Intern Med 1988; 108:7–13.
52. Hammond IW, Devereux RB, Alderman MH, et al. The prevalence and correlates of echocardiographic left ventricular hypertrophy among employed patients with uncomplicated hypertension. J Am Coll Cardiol 1986; 7:639–650.
53. Devereux RB, Alonso DR, Lutas EM, et al. Sensitivity of echocardiography for detection of left ventricular hypertrophy. In: Ter Keurs H, Schipperheyn JJ. Cardiac Left Ventricular Hypertrophy. The Hague: Martinus Nijhoff, 1983:16–37.
54. Savage DD, Drayer JIM, Henry WL, et al. Echocardiographic assessment of cardiac anatomy and function in hypertensive subjects. Circulation 1979; 59:623–632.
55. Drayer JI, Gardin J, Brewer DD, et al. Disparate relationships between blood pressure and left ventricular mass in patients with and without left ventricular hypertrophy. Hypertension 1987; 9(suppl II):II-61–II-64.
56. Messerli FH, Sundgaard-Riise K, Ventura HO, et al. Clinical and hemodynamic determinants of left ventricular dimensions. Arch Intern Med 1984; 144:447–481.
57. Baba S, Ozawa H, Nakamoto Y, et al. Enhanced blood pressure response to regular daily stress in urban hypertensive men. J Hypertens 1990; 8:647–655.
58. Devereux RB, Pickering TG, Harshfield GA, et al. Left ventricular hypertrophy in patients with hypertension: importance of blood pressure response to regularly recurring stress. Circulation 1983; 68:470–476.
59. Gosse P, Descrumeau GC, Roudaut R, et al. Left ventricular mass in normotensive subjects: importance of blood pressure response to activity. Am J Hypertens 1989; 2:78–80.
60. Mayet J, Shahi M, Hughes AD, Stanton AV, et al. Left ventricular structure and function in previously untreated hypertensive patients: the importance of blood pressure, the nocturnal blood pressure dip and heart rate. J Cardiovasc Risk 1995; 2:255–261.
61. Lemne C, Lindvall K, Georgiades A, Fredrikson M, de Faire U. Structural cardiac changes in relation to 24-h ambulatory blood pressure levels in borderline hypertension. J Intern Med 1995; 238:49–57.
62. White WB. Blood pressure load and target organ effects in patients with essential hypertension. J Hypertens 1991; 9(suppl 8):S39–S41.

63. Gatzka CD, Schmieder RE, Schobel HP, et al. Improved prediction of left ventricular mass from ambulatory blood pressure monitoring using average tension-time index. J Hypertens 1993; 11(suppl 5):S98–S99.

64. Roman MJ, Pickering TG, Pini R, Schwartz JE, Devereux RB. Prevalence and determinants of cardiac and vascular hypertrophy in hypertension. Hypertension 1995; 26:369–373.

65. Devereux RB, Lutas EM, Casale RN, et al. Standardization of M-mode echocardiographic left ventricular anatomic measurements. J Am Coll Cardiol 1984; 4:1222–1230.

66. Gardin JM, Henry WL, Savage DD, et al. Echocardiographic measurements in normal subjects: evaluation of an adult population without clinically apparent heart disease. J Clin Ultrasound 1979; 7:439–447.

67. Lindroos M, Kupari M, Heikkila J, Tilvis R. Echocardiographic evidence of left ventricular hypertrophy in a general aged population. Am J Cardiol 1994; 74:385–390.

68. Dannenberg AL, Levy D, Garrison RJ. Impact of age on echocardiographic left ventricular mass in a healthy population (the Framingham Study). Am J Cardiol 1989; 64:1066–1068.

69. Gardin JM, Siscovick D, Anton-Culver H, Lynch JC, et al. Sex, age, and disease affect echocardiographic left ventricular mass and systolic function in the free-living elderly: the Cardiovascular Health Study. Circulation 1995; 91:1739–1748.

70. Liebson PR, Grandits G, Prineas R, et al. Echocardiographic correlates of left ventricular structure among 844 mildly hypertensive men and women in the Treatment of Mild Hypertension Study (TOHMS). Circulation 1993; 87:476–486.

71. Gardin JM, Savage DD, Ware JH, Henry WL. Effect of age, sex, and body surface area on echocardiographic left ventricular wall mass in normal subjects. Hypertension 1987; 9:II-36–II-39.

72. Aurigemma GP, Gaasch WH. Gender differences in older patients with pressure-overload hypertrophy of the left ventricle. Cardiology 1995; 86:310–317.

73. Koenig H, Goldstone A, Lu CY. Testosterone-mediated sexual dimorphism in the rodent heart: Ventricular lysosomes, mitochondria, and cell growth are modulated by androgens. Circ Res 1982; 50:782–787.

74. Marcus L, Krause L, Weder AB, et al. Sex-specific determinants of increased left ventricular mass in the Tecumseh Blood Pressure Study. Circulation 1994; 90:928–936.

75. Liao Y, Cooper RS, Mensah GA, McGee DL. Left ventricular hypertrophy has a greater impact on survival in women than in men. Circulation 1995; 92:805–810.

76. de Simone G, Devereux RB, Daniels SR, Meyer RA. Gender differences in left ventricular growth. Hypertension 1995; 26:979–983.

77. Frohlich ED, Tarazi RC. Is arterial pressure the sole factor responsible for hypertensive cardiac hypertrophy? Part II. Am J Cardiol 1979; 44: 959–963.

78. Hypertension Detection and Follow-up Program Cooperative Group. Race, education and prevalence of hypertension. Am J Epidemiol 1977; 106:351–361.

79. McDonough JR, Garrison GE, Hames CG. Blood pressure and hypertensive disease among negros and whites. Ann Intern Med 1964; 61:208–228.

80. Liao Y, Cooper RS, McGee DL, Mensah GA, Ghali JK. The relative effects of left ventricular hypertrophy, coronary artery disease, and ventricular dysfunction on survival among black adults. JAMA 1995; 273:1592–1597.

81. Dunn FG, Oigman W, Sundgaard-Riise K, et al. Racial differences in cardiac adaptation to essential hypertension determined by echocardiographic indexes. J Am Coll Cardiol 1983; 1:1348–1351.

82. Messerli FH. Cardiopathy of obesity: a not-so-Victorian disease [editorial]. N Engl J Med 1986; 314:378–380.

83. Alpert MA, Lambert CR, Terry BE, Cohen MV, et al. Influence of left ventricular mass on left ventricular diastolic filling in normotensive morbid obesity. Am Heart J 1995; 130:1068–1073.

84. Grodzicki T, Gryglewska B, Czarnecka D, Kawecka-Jaszcz K, Kocemba J. Cadiac adaptation to obesity in elderly hypertensive patients. J Hypertens 1993; 11(suppl 5):S92–S93.

85. Himeno E, Nishino K, Nakashima Y, Kuroiwa A, Ikeda M. Weight reduction regresses left ventricular mass regardless of blood pressure level in obese subjects. Am Heart J 1996; 131:313–319.

86. Messerli FH, Nunez BD, Ventura HO, Snyder DW. Overweight and sudden death: increased ventricular ectopy in cardiopathy of obesity. Arch Intern Med 1987; 147:1725–1728.

87. Rasooly Y, Sasson Z, Gupta R. Relation between body fat distribution and left ventricular mass in men without structural heart disease or systemic hypertension. Am J Cardiol 1993; 71:1477–1479.

88. Intersalt Cooperative Research Group. INTERSALT: an international study of electrolyte excretion and blood pressure—results for 24 hour urinary sodium and potassium. Br Med J 1988; 297:319–328.

89. Sen S, Young DR. Role of sodium in modulation of myocardial hypertrophy in renal hypertensive rats. Hypertension 1986; 8:918–924.
90. Schmieder RE, Messerli FH, Garavaglia GF, et al. Dietary salt intake: a determinant for cardiac involvement in essential hypertension. Circulation 1988; 78:951–956.
91. Hammond IW, Devereux RB, Alderman MH, Laragh JH. Relation of blood pressure and body build to left ventricular mass in normotensive and hypertensive employed adults. J Am Coll Cardiol 1988; 12: 996–1004.
92. Schmieder RE, Grube E, Impelman V, Ruddel H, et al. Determinants of myocardial hypertrophy in mild essential hypertension: impact of dietary salt intake on left ventricular hypertrophy. Z Kardiol 1990; 79: 557–564.
93. Jula AM, Karanko HM. Effects on left ventricular hypertrophy of long-term nonpharmacological treatment with sodium restriction in mild-to-moderate essential hypertension. Circulation 1994; 89:1023–1031.
94. Daniels SD, Meyer RA, Loggie JM. Determinants of cardiac involvement in children and adolescents with essential hypertension [see comments]. Circulation 1990; 82:1243–1248.
95. Martell N, Rodrigo JL, Fernandez-Pinilla C, et al. Sodium intake and atrial natriuretic factor as determinants of left ventricular dimensions: the Torrejon Study. J Hypertens 1991; 9(suppl 6):S258–S259.
96. Woo KS, Wilson P, Gatland R, Mimran A. Dietary salt intake and arterial wall stiffness in elderly hypertension: determinants for left ventricular hypertrophy? [abstract]. J Hypertens 1994; 12(suppl):S80.
97. Du Cailar G, Ribstein J, Daures JP, Mimran A. Sodium and left ventricular mass in untreated hypertensive and normotensive subjects. Am J Physiol 1992; 263:H177–H181.
98. Kupari M, Koskinen P, Virolainen J. Correlates of left ventricular mass in a population sample aged 36 to 37 years: focus on lifestyle and salt intake. Circulation 1994; 89:1041–1050.
99. Langenfeld MR, Schmieder RE. Salt and left ventricular hypertrophy: what are the links? J Hum Hypertens 1995; 9:909–916.
100. Marmot MG, Elliot P, Shipley MJ, et al. Alcohol and blood pressure: the INTERSALT study. Br Med J 1994; 308:1263–1267.
101. Manolio TA, Levy D, Garrison RJ, et al. Relation of alcohol intake to left ventricular mass: The Framingham Study. J Am Coll Cardiol 1991; 17:717–721.
102. Palmer AJ, Fletcher AE, Bulpitt CJ, Beevers DG, Coles EC, Ledingham JGG, Petrie JC, Webster J, Dollery CT. Alcohol take and car-

diovascular mortality in hypertensive patients—a report from the Department of Health Hypertension Care Computing Project (DHCP). J Hypertens 1995; 13:957–964.

103. Schnall PL, Pieper C, Schwartz JE, et al. The relationship between "job strain," work place diastolic blood pressure, and left ventricular mass index: results of a case-control study. JAMA 1990; 263:1929–1935.

104. Frohlich ED. Hemodynamics and other determinants in development of left ventricular hypertrophy. Fed Proc 1983; 42:2709–2715.

105. Frohlich ED. The first Irvine H. Page lecture: the mosaic of hypertension: past present and future. J Hypertens 1988; 6(suppl):S2–S11.

106. Zhu YC, Zhu YZ, Spitznagel H, Gohlke P, Unger T. Substrate metabolism, hormone interaction, and angiotensin-converting enzyme inhibitors in left ventricular hypertrophy. Diabetes 1996; 45(suppl 1): S59–S65.

107. Costa CH, Batista MC, Moises VA, Kohlmann NB, et al. Serum insulin levels, 24-hour blood pressure profile, and left ventricular mass in nonobese hypertensive patients. Hypertension 1995; 26(6 pt 2): 1085–1088.

108. Diez J, Laviades C, Martinez E, Gil MJ, et al. Insulin-like growth factor binding proteins in arterial hypertension: relationship to left ventricular hypertrophy. J Hypertens 1995; 13:349–355.

109. Lind L, Andersson PE, Andren B, Hanni A, Lithell HO. Left ventricular hypertrophy in hypertension is associated with the insulin resistance metabolic syndrome. J Hypertens 1995; 13:433–438.

110. Duerr RL, Huang S, Miraliakbar HR, Clark R, et al. Insulin-like growth factor-1 enhances ventricular hypertrophy and function during the onset of experimental cardiac failure. J Clin Invest 1995; 95:619–627.

111. Yamazaki T, Komuro I, Kudoh S, Zou Y, Shiojima I, Mizuno T, Takano H, Hiroi Y, Ueki K, Tobe K, Kadowaki T, Nagai R, Yasaki Y. Angiotensin II partly mediates mechanical stress-induced cardiac hypertrophy. Circ Res 1995; 77:258–265.

112. Rostrup M, Smith G, Bjørnstad H, Westheim A, Stokland O, Eide I. Left ventricular mass and cardiovascular reactivity in young men. Hypertension 1994; 23(suppl I):I168–I171.

113. Linz W, Wiemer G, Gohlke P, Unger T, Scholkens BA. Contribution of kinins to the cardiovascular actions of angiotensin-converting enzyme inhibitors. Pharmacol Rev 1995; 47:25–49.

114. The SAVE Investigators: Pfeffer MA, Braumwald E, Moye LA, Basta L, Brown EJ Jr, Cuddy TE, Davis BR, Geltman EM, Goldman S,

Flaker GC, Klein M, Lamas GA, Packer M, Rouleau J, Rouleau JL, Rutheford J, Wertheimer JH, Hawkins CM. Effect of captopril on mortality and morbidity in patients with left ventricular dysfunction after myocardial infarction: results of the Survival and Ventricular Enlargement Trial. N Engl J Med 1992; 327:669–677.

115. Schmieder RE, Martus P, Klingbeil A. Reversal of left ventricular hypertrophy in essential hypertension: a meta-analysis of randomized double-blind studies. JAMA 1996; 275:1507–1513.

116. Liebson PR, Grandits GA, Dianzumba S, et al. Comparison of five antihypertensive monotherapies and placebo for change in left ventricular mass in patients receiving nutritional-hygienic therapy in the Treatment of Mild Hypertension Study (TOMHS). Circulation 1995; 91:698–706.

117. Sihm I, Schroeder AP, Aalkjaer C, Holm M, et al. Regression of media-to-lumen ratio of human subcutaneous arteries and left ventricular hypertrophy during treatment with an angiotensin-converting enzyme inhibitor-based regimen in hypertensive patients. Am J Cardiol 1995; 76:38E–40E.

118. Dzau VJ, Re RN. Tissue angiotensin system in cardiovascular medicine: a paradigm shift? Circulation 1994; 89:493–498.

119. Paul M, Bachmann J, Ganten D. The tissue renin-angiotensin systems in cardiovascular disease [review]. Trends Cardiovasc Med 1992; 2:94–99.

120. Dzau VJ. Local expression and pathophysiological role of renin angiotensin in the blood vessels and heart. In: Grobecker H, Heusch G, Strauer BE, eds. Angiotensin and the Heart. New York: Springer Verlag, 1993:1–14.

121. Dostol DE, Baker KM. Evidence for a role of an intracardiac renin-angiotensin system in normal and failing hearts. Trends Cardiovasc Med 1993; 3:67–74.

122. Linz W, Scholkens BA, Ganten D. Converting enzyme inhibition specifically prevents the development and induces regression of cardiac hypertrophy in rats. Clin Exp Hypertens 1989; 11:1325–1350.

123. The SOLVD Investigators. Effect of enalapril on survival in patients with reduced left ventricular ejection fractions and congestive heart failure. N Engl J Med 1991; 325:293–302.

124. Danser AHJ, Bax WA, Tavenier M, et al. Renin angiotensinogen and ACE in normal and failing human hearts [abstr]. Circulation 1993; 88 (suppl I):I-614.

125. Frohlich ED, Apstein C, Chobanian AV, Devereux RB, Dustan HP, Dzau V, Fauad-Tarazi F, Horan MJ, Marcus M, Massie B, Pfeffer

MA, Re RN, Rocella EJ, Savage D, Shub C. The heart in hypertension. N Engl J Med 1992; 327:998–1008.

126. Lindpaintner K, Lee M, Larson MG, Rao VS, et al. Absence of association or genetic linkage between the angiotensin-converting-enzyme gene and left ventricular mass. N Engl J Med 1996; 334:1023–1028.

127. Sporn MB, Roberts AB. Peptide growth factors are multifunctional. Nature 1988; 332:217–219.

128. Ikram H, Lynn KL, Bailey RR, Little PJ. Cardiovascular changes in chronic hemodialysis patients. Kidney Int 1983; 24:371–376.

129. Miach PJ, Dawborn JK, Louis WJ, McDonald IG. Left ventricular function in uremia: echocardiographic assessment in patients on maintenance dialysis. Clin Nephrol 1981; 15:259–263.

130. Harnett JD, Parfrey PS, Griffiths SM, Gault MH, Barre P, Guttman RD. Left ventricular hypertrophy in end-stage renal disease. Nephron 1988; 48:107–115.

131. Lindner A, Charra B, Sherrard DJ, Scribner BH. Accelerated atherosclerosis in prolonged maintenance hemodialysis. N Engl J Med 1974; 290:697–701.

132. London GM, Marchais SJ, Safar ME, Genest AF, Guerin AP, Metivier F, Chedid K, London AM. Aortic and large artery compliance in end-stage renal failure. Kidney Int 1990; 37:137–142.

133. Levin A, Singer J, Thompson CR, Ross H, Lewis M. Prevalent left ventricular hypertrophy in the predialysis population: identifying opportunities for intervention. Am J Kidney Dis 1996; 27:347–354.

134. Foley RN, Parfrey PS, Harnett JD, Kent GM, et al. The prognostic importance of left ventricular geometry in uremic cardiomyopathy. J Am Soc Nephrol 1995; 5:2024–2031.

135. de Wardener HE. The primary role of the kidney and salt intake in the etiology of essential hypertension: part I. Clin Sci 1990; 79:193–200.

136. Cordonnier D, Bayle F, Benhamon PY, Milongo R, Zaoui P, Maynard C, Halimi S. Future trends of management of renal failure in diabetics. Kidney Int 1993; 43(suppl):S8–S13.

137. Mignon F, Michel C, Mentre F, Viron B. Worldwide demographics and future trends of the management of renal failure in the elderly. Kidney Int 1993; 43(suppl):S18–S26.

138. Ibels LS, Alfrey AC, Huffer WE, Craswell PW, Anderson JT, Weil R III. Arterial calcification and pathology in uremic patients undergoing dialysis. Am J Med 1979; 66:790–796.

139. Laragh JH. The renin system and four lines of hypertension research: nephron heterogeneity, the calcium connection, the prorenin vaso-

dilator limb, and plasma renin and heart attack. Hypertension 1992; 20: 267–279.

140. Katz AM. Is angiotensin II a growth factor masquerading as vasopressor? Heart Dis Stroke 1992; 1:151–154.

141. Muirhead EE, Brooks B, Byers LW. Biologic differences between vasodilator prostaglandins and medullipin. Am J Med Sci 1992; 303:86–89.

142. Chaignon M, Chen WT, Tarazi RC, Bravo EL, Nakamoto S. Effect of hemodialysis on blood volume distribution and cardiac output. Hypertension 1981; 3:327–332.

143. Anderson CB, Codd JR, Graff RA, Groce MA, Harter HR, Newton WT. Cardiac failure and upper extremity arteriovenous dialysis fistula. Arch Intern Med 1976; 136:292–297.

144. Canziani ME, Cendoroglo Neto M, Saragoca MA, Cassiolato JL, et al. Hemodialysis versus continuous ambulatory peritoneal dialysis: effects on the heart. Artif Organs 1995; 19:241–244.

145. Silberberg JS, Rahal DP, Patton DR, Sniderman AD. Role of anemia in the pathogenesis of left ventricular hypertrophy in end-stage renal disease. Am J Cardiol 1989; 64:222–224.

146. Harnett JD, Kent GM, Foley RN, Parfrey PS. Cardiac function and hematocrit level. Am J Kidney Dis 1995; 25(4 suppl 1):S3–7.

147. Juric M, Rupcic V, Topuzovic N, Jakic M, et al. Haemodynamic changes and exercise tolerance in dialysis patients treated with erythropoietin. Nephrol Dialysis Transplant 1995; 10:1398–1404.

148. Baczinski R, Massry SG, Kohan R, Magott M, Saglikes Y, Brautbar N. Effect of parathyroid hormone on myocardial energy metabolism in rat. Kidney Int 1985; 27:718–725.

149. Bogin E, Massry SG, Harary I. Effect of parathyroid hormone on heart cells. J Clin Invest 1981; 67:1215–1227.

150. Besbas N, Saatci U, Ozkutlu S, Bakkaloglu A, et al. Effects of secondary hyperparathyroidism on cardiac function in pediatric patients on hemodialysis. Turk J Pediatr 1995; 37:299–304.

151. Mall G, Huther W, Schneider J, Lundin P, Ritz E. Diffuse intramyocardiocytic fibrosis in uraemic patients. Nephrol Dialysis Transplant 1990; 5:39–44.

152. Topol EJ, Traill TA, Tortuin NJ. Hypertensive hypertrophic cardiomyopathy of the elderly. N Engl J Med 1985; 312:277–283.

153. Sax FL, Brush JE, Cannon RO, et al. Impaired left ventricular filling in symptomatic compared to asymptomatic hypertensive patients [abstr]. J Am Coll Cardiol 1988; 11:81A.

154. Staiger J, Dickhuth HH, Keul J. Improvement of left ventricular diastolic function by endurance exercise: a contribution to rehabilitation after infarct? In: Franz IW, Mellerowicz H, Noack W, eds. Training and Sport for Prevention and Rehabilitation in the Technicized Environment. Berlin: Springer-Verlag, 1985:709.

155. Kannel WB, Castelli WP, McNamara PM, et al. Role of blood pressure in the development of congestive heart failure: the Framingham Study. N Engl J Med 1972; 287:781–787.

156. de Simone D, Devereux RB, Roman MJ, et al. Assessment of left ventricular function by the midwall fractional fiber shortening/end systolic stress relation in human hypertension. J Am Coll Cardiol 1994; 23:1444–1451.

157. de Simone G, Devereux RB, Koren MJ, Mensah GA, et al. Midwall left ventricular mechanics: an independent predictor of cardiovascular risk in arterial hypertension. Circulation 1996; 93:259–265.

158. Maron BJ, Ferrans FJ, Roberts WC. Ultrastructural features of degenerated cardiac muscle cells in patients with cardiac hypertrophy. Am J Pathol 1975; 79:387–434.

159. Aurigemma GP, Gaasch WH, McLaughlin M, McGinn R, et al. Reduced left ventricular systolic pump performance and depressed myocardial contractile function in patients >65 years of age with normal ejection fraction and a high relative wall thickness. Am J Cardiol 1995; 76:702–705.

160. Mueller TM, Marcus ML, Kerber RE, et al. Effect of renal hypertension and left ventricular hypertrophy on the coronary circulation in dogs. Circ Res 1978; 42:543–549.

161. O'Keefe DD, Hoffman JIE, Cheitlin R, et al. Coronary blood flow in experimental canine left ventricular hypertrophy. Circ Res 1978; 43:43–51.

162. Schroeder AP, Brysting B, Sogaard P, Pedersen OL. Silent myocardial ischemia in untreated essential hypertensives. Blood Press 1995; 4: 97–104.

163. Vassalli G, Kaufmann P, Villari B, Jakob M, et al. Reduced epicardial coronary vasodilator capacity in patients with left ventricular hypertrophy. Circulation 1995; 91:2916–2923.

164. Strauer BE. Left ventricular wall stress and hypertrophy. In: Messerli FH, ed. The Heart and Hypertension. New York: Yorke Medical Books, 1987:153.

165. Strauer BE. Myocardial oxygen consumption in chronic heart disease: role of wall stress, hypertrophy and coronary reserve. Am J Cardiol 1979; 44:730–740.

166. Tomanek RJ, Palmer PH, Pfeiffer GL, et al. Morphometry of canine coronary arteries, arterioles and capillaries during hypertension and left ventricular hypertrophy. Circ Res 1986; 58:38–46.
167. Marcus ML, Harrison DG, Chilian WM, et al. Alterations in the coronary circulation in the hypertrophied ventricles. Circulation 1987; 75 (suppl 1):I-19–I-25.
168. Pichard AD, Gorlin R, Smith H, et al. Coronary flow studies in patients with left ventricular hypertrophy of the hypertensive type: evidence for an impaired coronary vascular reserve. Am J Cardiol 1981; 47:547–554.
169. Strauer BE. Comparative analysis of cardiac function, geometry, energetics and coronary reserve in hypertensive heart disease. Nephron 1987; 47(suppl 1):76–86.
170. Scheler S, Motz W, Strauer BE. Transient myocardial ischemia in hypertensive heart disease. Z Kardiol 1989; 78:197–203.
171. Messerli FH, Ventura HO, Elizardi DJ, et al. Hypertension and sudden death: increased ventricular ectopic activity in left ventricular hypertrophy. Am J Med 1984; 77:18–22.
172. Messerli FH, Nunez BD, Nunez MM, et al. Hypertension and sudden death: disparate effects of calcium entry blocker and diuretic therapy on cardiac dysrhythmias. Arch Intern Med 1989; 149(suppl 6):1263–1267.
173. McLenachan JM, Henderson E, Morris KI, et al. Ventricular arrhythmias in patients with hypertensive left ventricular hypertrophy. N Engl J Med 1987; 317:787–792.
174. Bikkina M, Larson MG, Levy D. Asymptomatic ventricular arrhythmias and mortality risk in subjects with left ventricular hypertrophy. J Am Coll Cardiol 1993; 22:1111–1116.
175. Almendral J, Villacastin JP, Arenal A, Tercedor L, et al. Evidence favoring the hypothesis that ventricular arrhythmias have prognostic significance in left ventricular hypertrophy secondary to systemic hypertension. Am J Cardiol 1995; 76:60D–63D.
176. Ghali JK, Kadakia S, Cooper RS, et al. Impact of left ventricular hypertrophy on ventricular arrhythmias in the absence of coronary artery disease. J Am Coll Cardiol 1991; 17:1277–1282.
177. Opherk D, Mall G, Zebe M, et al. Reduction of coronary reserve: a mechanism for angina pectoris in patients with arterial hypertension and normal coronary arteries. Circulation 1984; 69:1–7.
178. Szlachcic J, Tubau J, O'Kelly B, et al. What is the role of silent coronary artery and left ventricular hypertrophy in the genesis of ventricular

arrhythmias in men with essential hypertension? J Am Coll Cardiol 1992; 19:803–808.

179. Weber KT, Janicki JS, Shroff SG, et al. Collagen compartment and remodeling in the pressure overloaded left ventricle. J Appl Cardiol 1988; 3:37.

180. Mandawat MK, Wallbridge DR, Pringle SD, Ruyami AA, et al. Heart rate variability of left ventricular hypertrophy. Br Heart J 1995; 73: 139–144.

181. Palatini P, Maraglino G, Accurso V, Sturaro M, et al. Impaired left ventricular filling hypertensive left ventricular hypertrophy as a marker of the presence of an arrhythmogenic substrate. Br Heart J 1995; 73:258–262.

182. Devereux RD, Dahlöf B. Criteria for an informative trial of left ventricular hypertrophy regression. J Hum Hypertens 1994; 8:735–739.

7

Uremic Cardiomyopathy

**Eberhard Ritz, Ute Schwarz, Michael Rambausek,
and Kerstin Amann**   Ruperto Carola University, Heidelberg,
Germany

SUMMARY

Cardiac mortality in dialysed patients is higher than in any other high
risk population—equivalent to that in survivors of myocardial infarction. Undoubtedly the high prevalence of coronary disease is an
important causal factor. Nevertheless, ischemic heart disease is seen
even in patients with patent coronary arteries. Apparently the evolution of heart disease is particularly severe in dialysed patients.

   Noncoronary factors compromising heart function in the renal
patient include left ventricular hypertrophy (which cannot be explained
exclusively as a consequence of hypertension), cardiac fibrosis (which
interferes with cardiac compliance and electrical stability of the
heart), and disturbances of the cardiac microcirculation (which interferes with coronary reserve and reduces ischemia tolerance).

   All these factors reduce ischemia tolerance. Raising hemoglobin concentrations is therefore a rational therapeutic strategy in the
renal patient with heart disease.

EPIDEMIOLOGY OF CARDIAC DEATH IN DIALYSED PATIENTS

Cardiac death accounts for approximately 50% of all fatalities in the dialysis population, according to the U.S. Renal Data System (1) and the registry of the European Dialysis Transplant Association (EDTA) (2). The EDTA Registry Report documented that, in any subgroup— e.g., males or females, or residents of high-cardiac-risk vs. low-cardiac-risk countries—the probability of cardiac death is higher in the dialysis population by a factor of approximately 20. Table 1 illustrates how dramatically increased the cardiac risk in renal patients actually is compared to non-renal patients (3). It shows that in the non-diabetic patient on renal replacement therapy, the risk of death from myocardial infarction is similar to that of the survivor of myocardial infarction in the ISIS-2 trial. It is higher still in the diabetic patient on renal replacement therapy.

This excessive cardiac risk of the dialysis patient, which is not well appreciated by nonnephrologists, calls for an explanation. There is no doubt that coronary artery disease is common in the dialysis population. This is not surprising in view of the cumulation of risk factors such as hypertension and dyslipidemia, and perhaps also of

Table 1   Cardiovascular Mortality in Dialysed Patients

MRFIT screenee cohort, 10-year follow-up	
($n = 347,978$)	
Hypertensive diabetic	10/1000 pts/years *total* mortality
Hypertensive nondiabetic	3/1000 pts/years
ISIS-2 postmyocardial infarction trial placebo group	
($n = 1241$), 4-year follow-up	26/1000 pts/years *MI* mortality
U.K. end-stage renal failure patients commencing renal replacement therapy, 1981–1985	
($n = 6742$), 5-year follow-up	
Diabetic	65/1000 pts/years *MI* mortality
Nondiabetic	20/1000 pts/years *MI* mortality

Source: Courtesy of Professor Raine.

some unconventional risk factors such as cumulation of AGE peptides and hyperhomocysteinemia. Nevertheless, postmortem studies (4,5) showed that the prevalence of coronary heart disease is "only" around 30%—at least among non-diabetic patients—and this estimate is supported by studies in which dialysis patients were subjected to coronarography (6,7). The latter studies are limited in scope, since, for obvious reasons, coronarography was not administered in a random fashion. Rostand et al. (8) clearly described the occurrence of angina pectoris and ischemic heart disease in dialysis patients who had patent coronary arteries. It is therefore obvious that—apart from the undoubted coronary problems—noncoronary factors contribute to the high incidence of cardiac events in the dialysis population. Whether the final result (9) should be designated "uremic cardiomyopathy" is more a semantic than a scientific problem.

LEFT VENTRICULAR HYPERTROPHY

The careful and elegant studies of Parfrey et al. (10,11) clearly documented the enormous prevalence of left ventricular hypertrophy (LVH) in the dialysis population: At the time of the start of dialysis, approximately 70% of the patients have LVH, and the proportion increases further with increasing duration of dialysis treatment. Both eccentric and concentric hypertrophy are seen; this may depend on the relative contributions of increased preload and afterload.

In patients with primary hypertension, LVH is a potent predictor of ventricular arrhythmia and cardiac death, independent of blood pressure (12,13). This is also the case in the dialysis population (14), as illustrated by the study of Silberberg et al. (14) (Figure 1).

The question arises whether LVH is merely the consequence of increased blood pressure or whether other factors contribute to its genesis (9). In normotensive dialysis patients, Hüting et al. (15) undertook a longitudinal study and noted that posterior wall thickness and septal thickness increased progressively with time. In agreement with such evidence of increased LV mass independent of hypertension is the observation of Rambausek et al. (16) in subtotally nephrectomized rats; LVH was increased even when the animals were subjected to effective α- and β-blockade, reduction of arterial

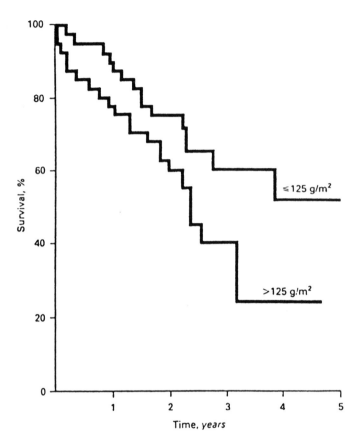

Figure 1 Left ventricular hypertrophy reduces actuarial survival in dialysis patients. Cumulative survival according to echocardiographic left ventricular hypertrophy defined as LVMI > 125 g/m², i.e., above the 95th centile of the normal population. (After Ref. 14.)

blood pressure (including by ACE inhibitor treatment), and reduction of hypervolemia by furosemide treatment. It goes without saying that one important contributing factor is anemia. This was most elegantly documented by studies that showed that LV mass was significantly reduced, but not completely normalized, following treatment with rhEPO (17–20).

Additional Factors That May Contribute to LVH

Although a number of possible other factors must be considered (9), we wish to draw attention to the much neglected observation of London et al. (21) that aortic elasticity is significantly diminished in dialysis patients. This abnormality increases with duration of dialysis. Diminished aortic elasticity must increase impedance and increase the kinetic work of the heart. Such increased peak systolic stress will undoubtedly contribute to LVH. Reduced aortic elasticity is explained, at least in part, by reduced aortic elastic fiber content (Figure 2), as shown in experimental studies (22).

The Possible Consequences of LVH in Uremic Patients

LVH is known to predispose to ventricular arrhythmia (12,13). It also alters the LV strain–stress relationship. LV compliance is impaired as a result of LV hypertrophy, and an important consequence thereof is blood-pressure instability on dialysis (23,24). Ruffmann et al. (23) showed that the LV mass:volume ratio was more abnormal in patients with repeated intradialytic hypotensive episodes than in patients without (Figure 3); this was accompanied by an abnormal transmitral inflow pattern as studied by Doppler ultrasound technique.

CARDIAC FIBROSIS

In renal patients, cardiac fibrosis was described decades ago (25), but these early observations were completely forgotten. Both experimental (26) and clinical (27) studies by the Heidelberg group documented that uremia causes marked fibrosis of the cardiac interstitium that is not explained by blood-pressure elevation and LV hypertrophy (Figure 4). It is associated with selective activation of interstitial cells as documented by stereological measurements (Table 2) and immunohistochemical staining for cytokines and growth factors (9). It is of interest that PTH appears to be permissive for the genesis of cardiac fibrosis in renal failure (28).

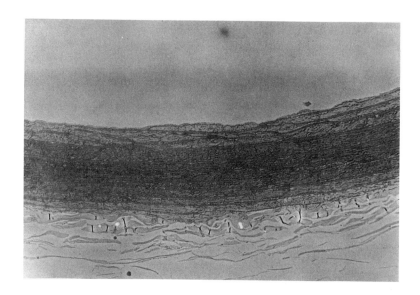

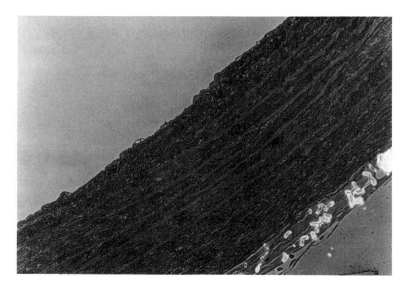

Figure 2 (Top) Aorta of a sham-operated control animal. Semithin section, methylen blue and basic fuchsin. Magnification: 1:105. (Bottom) Aorta of a subtotally nephrectomized rat 8 weeks after operation. Note wall thickening of the aortic media with increased extracellular matrix and hyperplasia of vascular smooth muscle cells. In parallel, the relative contents of elastic fibers are markedly reduced. Semithin section, methylen blue and basic fuchsin. Magnification: 1:105.

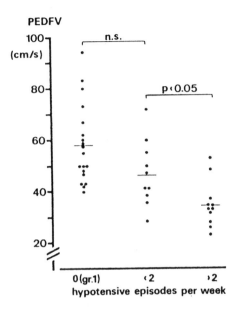

Figure 3   Left ventricular diastolic filling characteristics in dialysis patients with no intradialytic hypotension, either infrequent or frequent intradialytic hypotensive episodes. PEDFV = peak velocity or early diastolic filling. (After Ref. 23.)

Table 2   Selective Enlargement of Interstitial, But Not Endothelial, Cells in the Heart of Uremic Animals

Volumes (μ^3)	NX ($n = 7$)	CO ($n = 7$)
Endothelial cells		
Cytoplasm	119 ± 58	146 ± 87
Nuclei	106 ± 19	100 ± 13
Interstitial cells		
Cytoplasm	425 ± 348	85 ± 67[a]
Nuclei	130 ± 39	98 ± 14[b]

[a] $p < 0.01$.
[b] $p < 0.05$.
Source: After Ref. 26.

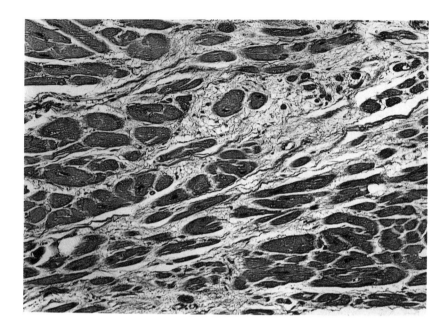

Figure 4 Uremic cardiomyopathy. Note hypertrophy of cardiomyocytes and diffuse interstitial fibrosis. Paraffin section, HE stain. Magnification: 1:450.

Cardiac fibrosis in uremia is not a replacement type of fibrosis, i.e., substitution of scar tissue for necrotic parenchyma; its extension does also not correspond to vascular territories. It is a primary type of cardiac fibrosis (29) that results from direct activation of interstitial cells and may have considerable functional consequences: altered LV compliance, altered strain–stress relationship, and electrical instability, as discussed in detail elsewhere (9).

CORONARY PERFUSION (CORONARY RESERVE)

The occurrence of angina pectoris despite patent coronaries (8,30) is reminiscent of syndrome X, characterized by angina pectoris in

Table 3 Length Density (LV) of Capillaries in the Hearts of Uremic Animals

	Controls (n = 7)	Uremia (n = 8)	Goldblatt HT LV weight-matched (n = 10)
LV (mm/mm^3)	3364 ± 183	2485 ± 264[a]	3155 ± 312

[a] $p < 0.01$ vs. controls.
Source: After Ref. 32.

hypertensive patients who have patent coronary arteries but diminished coronary reserve upon investigation with dipyridamol. The question arises whether structural abnormalities of the cardiac microvasculature contribute to diminished coronary perfusion reserve in renal patients. In the LV of subtotally nephrectomized rats, stereological measurements showed a reduction in capillary density (32) as well as altered wall structure of arterioles (22). As shown in Table 3, the length density of capillaries (i.e., conceptually, the length of all capillaries added one to another that are contained within one volume element of myocardial tissue) is significantly diminished in the LV of uremic rats compared to control rats or hypertensive rats. Apparently, growth of capillaries does not keep pace with the growth of cardiomyocytes, so hypertrophic oxygen demanding parenchyma outgrows its capillary supply. As a consequence, cardiac tissue is at greater risk of critical hypoxia.

Furthermore (Table 4), the wall thickness of arterioles is increased in the heart of uremic animals, even when hypertension is reversed by antihypertensive medication (22). According to the concepts of Folkow, contraction of vascular smooth-muscle cells in the walls of hypertrophied vessels with reduced lumen will translate into a greater increment of vascular resistance. Wall-thickening does not necessarily imply increased resistance to flow under basal conditions, but it will certainly interfere with the ability of the vessels to adequately dilate in response to increased oxygen demand. Diminished coronary reserve in syndrome X is accompanied by similar arteriolar wall-thickening (33).

Table 4 Wall/Lumen Ratio of Cardiac Arterioles in Subtotally Nephrectomized Rats With and Without Antihypertensive Treatment (Hydralazine Plus Furosemide)

	Systolic blood pressure (mm Hg)	Wall thickness (μm)			
		Intramyocardial arterioles	Media of aorta	Mesenteric arteries	Mesenteric arteries
Untreated controls ($n = 10$)	110 ± 13.3	1.7 ± 0.27	103 ± 14	10.8 ± 1.53	3.36 ± 1.01
Treated controls ($n = 9$)	99 ± 8.1	1.61 ± 0.13	110 ± 15	10.1 ± 3.4	3.7 ± 0.69
Untreated SNX ($n = 8$)	132 ± 20.7	2.33 ± 0.35	138 ± 29	15.5 ± 2.82	5.22 ± 0.69
Treated SNX ($n = 8$)	103 ± 13	2.15 ± 0.19	130 ± 19	15.2 ± 3.45	5.57 ± 1.97

x ± SD. Significant differences for all structural parameters between treated SNX and treated controls.
Source: After Ref. 22.

It is obvious that factors other than impaired vascular structures may also interfere with ischemia tolerance. Observations that are relevant in this context include diminished stability of phosphocreatine concentrations in the isolated perfused Langendorf preparation of uremic animals (34) and diminished insulin-dependent glucose uptake (35,36) accompanied by impaired availability of insulin-sensitive glucose-transporting molecules (Glut-4).

PERSPECTIVES

Obviously a number of factors merge in uremia to expose the heart to an increased risk of ischemia. The disturbed supply–demand relationship—increased oxygen demand (hypertension, anemia, etc.) in the presence of diminished oxygen supply (coronary atheroma, flow restriction on the arteriolar and capillary level of the vascular bed)—is aggravated by metabolic abnormalities (nucleotide stability, regulation of intracellular Ca^{2+}, glucose uptake) and interferes with the ability of the heart to resist ischemia.

One factor that will definitely reduce such ischemia intolerance is reversal of anemia by rhEPO. Although no controlled evidence is available, anecdotal observations of Wizemann et al. (37) show impressive amelioration of the sequelae of cardiac ischemia following partial correction of anemia.

REFERENCES

1. US Renal Data System. Causes of Death, Annual Data Report. Bethesda, MD: National Institute of Diabetes and Digestive and Kidney Diseases, National Institutes of Health, 1995; 14:79–90.
2. European Transplantation and Dialysis Association. Report on Management of Renal Failure in Europe, XXII, 1991. Nephrol Dialysis Transplant 1995; 10(suppl 5):12.
3. Neaton JD, Kuller L, Stamler J, Wentworth DN. Impact of systolic and diastolic blood pressure on cardiovascular mortality. In: Laragh JH, Brenner BM, eds. Hypertension: Pathophysiology, Diagnosis and Management. 2nd ed. New York: Raven Press, 1995:127–144.
4. Clyne N, Lins LE, Kenneth Pehrsson S. Occurrence and significance of heart disease in uremia. Scand J Urol Nephrol 1986; 20:307–311.
5. Ansari A, Kaupke CJ, Vaziri ND, Miller R, Barbari A. Cardiac pathology in patients with end-stage renal disease maintained on hemodialysis. Int J Artific Organs 1993; 16:31–36.
6. Ikram H, Lynn KL, Bailey RR, Little PJ. Cardiovascular changes in chronic hemodialysis patients. Kidney Int 1983; 24:371–376.
7. Hässler R, Höfling B, Castro L, Gurland HJ, Hillebrand G, Land W, Erdmann E. Koronare Herzkrankheit und Herzklappenerkarnkungen bei Patienten mit terminaler Niereninsuffizienz. Deutsche Medizinische Wochenschrift 1987; 18:714–718.
8. Rostand SG, Kirk KA, Rutsky EA. Dialysis-associated ischemic heart disease: insights from coronary angiography. Kidney Int 1984; 25:653–659.
9. Amann K, Ritz E. Cardiac structure and function in renal disease. Curr Opin Nephrol Hypertension 1996; 5:102–106.
10. Parfrey PS, Harnett JD, Griffiths SM, Taylor R, Hand J, King A, Barre PE. The clinical course of left ventricular hypertrophy. Nephron 1990; 55:114–120.
11. Parfrey PS, Griffiths SM, Harnett JD, Taylor R, King A, Hand J, Barre PE. Outcome of congestive heart failure, dilated cardiomyopathy, hypertrophic hyperkinetic disease, and ischemia heart disease in dialysis patients. Am J Nephrol 1990; 10:213–221.

12. Casale PN, Devereux RB, Milner M, Zullo G, Harshfield GA, Pickering TG, Laragh JH. Value of echocardiographic left ventricular mass in predicting cardiovascular morbid events in hypertensive men. Ann Intern Med 1986; 105:173–178.
13. Levy D, Anderson KM, Savage DD, Balkus SA, Kannel WB, Castelli WP. Risk of ventricular arrhythmias in left ventricular hypertrophy: The Framingham Heart Study. Am J Cardiol 1987; 60:560–565.
14. Silberberg JS, Barre PE, Prichard SS, Sniderman AD. Impact of left ventricular hypertrophy on survival in end-stage renal disease. Kidney Int 1989; 36:286–290.
15. Hüting J, Kramer W, Reitinger J, Kühn K, Wizemann V, Schütterle G. Cardiac structure and function in continuous ambulatory peritoneal dialysis: influence of blood purification and hypercirculation. Am Heart J 1990; 119:344–348.
16. Rambausek M, Ritz E, Mall G, Mehls O, Katus H. Myocardial hypertrophy in rats with renal insufficiency. Kidney Int 1985; 28:775–782.
17. Macdougall IC, Lewis NP, Saunders MJ, Cochlin DL, Davies ME, Hutton RD, Fox KAA, Coles GA, Williams JD. Long-term cardiorespiratory effects of amelioration of renal anaemia by erythropoietin. Lancet 1990; 335:489–493.
18. London GM, Zins B, Pannier B, Naret C, Berthelot JM, Jacquot C, Safar M, Drucke TB. Vascular changes in hemodialysis patients in response to recombinant human erythropoetin. Kidney Int 1989; 36:878–882.
19. Cannella G, Paoletti E, Delfino R, Peloso G, Molinari S, Traverso GB. Regression of left ventricular hypertrophy in hypertensive dialyzed uremic patients on long-term antihypertensive therapy. Kidney Int 1993; 44:881–886.
20. Silberberg JS, Racine N, Barre P, Sniderman AD. Regression of left ventricular hypertrophy in dialysis patients following correction of anemia with recombinant human erythropoietin. Can J Cardiol 1990; 6(1):1–4.
21. London GM, Marchais SJ, Safar ME, Genest AF, Guerin AP, Metivier F, Chedid K, London AM. Aortic and large artery compliance in end-stage renal failure. Kidney Int 1990; 37:137–142.
22. Amann K, Neusüß R, Ritz E, Irzyniec T, Wiest G, Mall G. Changes of vascular architecture independent of blood pressure in experimental uremia. Am J Hypertension 1995; 8:409–417.

23. Ruffmann K, Mandelbaum A, Bommer J, Schmidli M, Ritz E. Doppler echocardiographic findings in dialysis patients. Nephrol Dialysis Transplant 1990; 5:426–431.
24. Ritz E, Ruffmann K, Rambausek M, Mall G, Schmidli M. Dialysis hypotension: is it related to diastolic left ventricular malfunction? Nephrol Dialysis Transplant 1987; 2:293–297.
25. Rössle H. Über die serösen Entzündungen der Organe. [On the serous inflammation of the organs.] Virchows Archiv 1943; 311:252–284.
26. Mall G, Rambausek M, Neumeister A, Kollmar S, Vetterlein F, Ritz E. Myocardial interstitial fibrosis in experimental uremia: implications for cardiac compliance. Kidney Int 1988; 33:804–811.
27. Mall G, Huther W, Schneider J, Lundin P, Ritz E. Diffuse intermyocardiocytic fibrosis in uremic patients. Nephrol Dialysis Transplant 1990; 5:39–44.
28. Amann K, Wiest G, Klaus G, Ritz E, Mall G. The role of parathyroid-hormone in the genesis of interstitial cell activation in uremia. J Am Soc Nephrol 1994; 4:1814–1819.
29. Weber KT, Sun Y, Tyagi SC, Cleutjens JP. Collagen network of the myocardium: function, structural remodeling and regulatory mechanisms. J Molec Cell Cardiol 1994; 26:279–292.
30. Roig E, Betriu A, Castaner A, Magrina J, Sanz G, Navarra Lopez F. Disabling angina pectoris with normal coronary arteries in patients undergoing hemodialysis. Am J Med 1981; 71:437–444.
31. Opherk D, Mall G, Zebe H, Schwarz F, Weihe E, Manthey J, Kübler W. Reduction of coronary reserve: a mechanism for angina pectoris in patients with arterial hypertension and normal coronary arteries. Circulation 1984; 69:1–7.
32. Amann K. Wiest G, Zimmer G, Gretz N, Ritz E, Mall G. Reduced capillary density in the myocardium of uremic rats: a stereological study. Kidney Int 1992; 42:1079–1085.
33. Schwarzkopff B, Motz W, Frenzel H, Vogt M, Knauer S, Strauer BE. Structural and functional alterations of the intramyocardial coronary arterioles in patients with arterial hypertension. Circulation 1993; 88: 993–1003.
34. Raine AEG, Seymour AML, Roberts AFC, Radda GK, Ledingham JGG. Impairment of cardiac function and energetics in experimental renal failure. J Clin Invest 1993; 92:2934–2940.
35. Ritz E, Koch M. Hypertension as risk factors for renal patients. Am J Kidney Dis 1993; 21(suppl 2):113–118.

36. Matthias S, Hönack C, Rösen P, Zebe H, Ritz E. Glucose uptake and expression of glucose transporters in the heart of uremic rats. J Am Soc Nephrol 1995; 6:1023.
37. Wizemann V, Schäfer R, Kramer W. Follow-up of cardiac changes induced by anemia compensation in normotensive hemodialysis patients with left-ventricular hypertrophy. Nephron 1993; 64:202–206.

8

Microalbumin and Cardiovascular Risk in Hypertension

Bhuwnesh Agrawal   Boehringer Mannheim GmbH, Mannheim, Germany

Friedrich C. Luft   Franz Volhard Clinic at the Max Delbrück Center for Molecular Medicine, Humboldt University of Berlin, Berlin, Germany

INTRODUCTION

Microalbuminuria (MAU) is associated with the development of clinical proteinuria, chronic renal failure, and premature cardiovascular mortality in patients with insulin-dependent, type I diabetes mellitus (1). MAU is also associated with cardiovascular morbidity and mortality in patients with non-insulin-dependent, type II diabetes mellitus (2). Furthermore, MAU has received increasing attention as a risk indicator in hypertensive patients without diabetes mellitus (3–7). However, the numbers of subjects in these investigations were generally small. The clinical significance of MAU in hypertensive patients in a practice setting remains uncertain. The purpose of our survey was to test the implications of MAU in nondiabetic hypertensive patients in a practice setting. Since practical utility and cost-consciousness are both important issues, we used an inexpensive immunoassay test strip, which was employed by the physicians and the patients. We found that MAU had important risk implications for these patients.

METHODS

We recruited general practitioners who were willing to enroll hypertensive patients in their practices into the study. All patients with treated or untreated hypertension in general practices throughout Germany were eligible; recruitment was conducted after due approval by an ethics committee and after informed consent was obtained. Details are outlined elsewhere (7). The frequency of concomitant diseases or complicating conditions was assessed by history, by reviewing medical records, and by conducting a physical examination. Myocardial infarction was diagnosed on the basis of the electrocardiogram or clear-cut evidence such as documented earlier events with enzyme determinations from prior medical records. Coronary artery disease was defined as angina pectoris requiring antianginal medication. Stroke was assessed on the basis of the physical examination or the patient's prior medical record. Peripheral occlusive vascular disease was assessed historically in terms of prior operations and clinically in terms of claudication, by physical examination, or by appropriate noninvasive or invasive visualization. These diagnoses were not made according to preset criteria but according to each practitioner's opinion. Blood-pressure measurements were conducted noninvasively in the sitting position by the Riva-Rocci method in triplicate in the physician's office.

Routine laboratory tests included total serum cholesterol, triglycerides, serum creatinine, and blood-sugar concentrations. Renal insufficiency (unusual because patients with proteinuria were excluded) was defined as creatinine concentration >1.8 mg/dl. The presence of hypertensive retinopathy was defined as $\geq +2$ (2 = arteriolar narrowing and arteriovenous nicking abnormalities). Diabetes mellitus was excluded by 2-hour postprandial glucose values or oral glucose-tolerance test. Hyperlipidemia was defined as elevated age-adjusted total serum cholesterol (>225 mg/dl for patients aged 30–39 years; >245 mg/dl for those aged 40–49 years; and >265 mg/dl for those aged >50 years), elevated triglycerides (>160 mg/dl), or both. Left ventricular hypertrophy (LVH) was defined as positive by either electrocardiogram (Sokolow and Lyon) or with echocardiographic criteria when available. Thus, the frequency of LVH was probably underestimated in the study.

MAU (defined as 20–200 mg/L) was determined by the Micral-Test (Boehringer Mannheim GmbH, Mannheim, Germany). The Micral-Test is an immunoassay specific for albumin (8). The test strip consists of a series of reagent pads. Urine is drawn by a chromatographic process and is buffered to an alkaline pH. The albumin in the urine binds to a soluble conjugate of albumin antibody and β-galactosidase. Excess albumin is immobilized and removed from the sample so that only albumin bound to the antibody–enzyme complex may react with the color pad. The substrate is chlorophenol red-galactoside, which is split by the enzyme. The color intensity after precisely 5 minutes is then compared to a reference chart. There are five color blocks, corresponding to 0, 10, 20, 50, and 100 mg/L.

The test was conducted three times on consecutive days on the first morning urine by the patients after they had been instructed in the test. The morning urine was selected to standardize the specimens in terms of the maximum concentration that would increase the yield of detected MAU. The patients were asked to read the test after 5 minutes (a stopwatch was provided) and then enter the values on diary cards, which were returned to the physician. MAU was considered positive, if *two of the three tests* had a reading of ≥20 mg/L. Of 11,920 patients enrolled, 11,343 had three MAU tests (95.2%); these patients were included in the analysis. The demographic data are shown in Table 1. Of these patients, 2744 had blood-pressure values under adequate control (<140/95 mm Hg). The duration of hypertension, duration, and treatment and systolic and diastolic blood pressures were slightly higher in the MAU group than in non-MAU patients. Furthermore, MAU was slightly more common ($p < 0.05$) in men (32%) than in women (28%).

Table 1   Demographic Data for the Patients

Parameter	All patients	MAU	non-MAU	$p <$
Number	11,343 (100%)	3405 (30%)	7939 (70%)	0.0001
Age (yr)	57.3 ± 0.1	58.4 ± 0.2	56.8 ± 0.1	0.002
Weight (kg)	78.8 ± 0.1	79.5 ± 0.2	78.5 ± 0.1	0.001
Height (cm)	170 ± 0.2	170 ± 0.1	170 ± 0.1	NS
Male:female ratio	50.9:49.1	53.3:46.7	49.9:50.1	0.0001
Duration of hypertension (mo)	69.1 ± 68.2	74.7 ± 1.2	66.7 ± 0.75	0.0001
Duration of antihyper- tensive treatment (mo)	65.9 ± 0.6	70.6 ± 1.1	63.8 ± 0.7	0.0001
Systolic blood pressure (mm Hg)	165.9 ± 0.2	170.1 ± 0.32	164.1 ± 0.2	0.0001
Diastolic blood pressure (mm Hg)	98.4 ± 0.1	100.5 ± 0.2	97.5 ± 0.1	0.0001
Heart rate (bpm)	77.5 ± 0.1	78.4 ± 0.2	77.1 ± 0.1	0.0001
Serum creatinine (mg/dl)	0.95 ± 0.0	0.97 ± 0.0	0.93 ± 0.0	0.0001

RESULTS

Table 2 shows the frequency of concomitant diseases in the patient groups. As can be observed, patients with MAU had higher rates of all concomitant diseases or complicating conditions with the exception of renal insufficiency (defined as serum creatinine >1.8 mg/dl), which was quite low in the sample population, since patients with renal insufficiency generally have overt proteinuria. Hypertensive retinopathy and LVH were 70% more common in patients with positive MAU than in those negative for MAU. For peripheral vascular disease and myocardial infarction, the frequency was almost 50% higher in MAU patients than in non-MAU patients. The rates of coronary artery disease and stroke were approximately 40% higher in the MAU group than in the non-MAU group.

The multiple stepwise regression analysis with MAU as the dependent variable showed that MAU depended on the following factors in the order shown: systolic BP > presence of retinopathy >

Table 2 Frequency of MAU in Concomitant Diseases or Complicating
Conditions in MAU and Non-MAU Patients

Disease/risk factor	All patients (%)	MAU (%)	Non-MAU (%)	p <
Hyperlipidemia	53.8	57.4	52.2	0.001
Coronary artery disease	25.0	31.0	22.4	0.001
Hypertensive retinopathy	18.6	26,.0	15.1	0.001
Left ventricular hypertrophy	17.0	24.0	13.8	0.001
Peripheral occlusive vascular disease	5.6	7.3	4.9	0.001
Myocardial infarction	5.4	7.0	4.0	0.001
Stroke	4.7	5.8	4.2	0.001
Creatinine concentration >1.8 mg/dl	0.6	0.6	0.6	—

presence of coronary artery disease > diastolic BP > heart rate > LVH
(all $p < 0.0001$) > presence of peripheral vascular disease ($p < 0.0005$)
> male gender ($p < 0.05$). We also performed a multiple stepwise
regression analysis with each of the concomitant diseases or complicating factors as the dependent variable. MAU was an independent
and significant variable for each of the conditions. With the exception of stroke ($p < 0.05$), myocardial infarction ($p < 0.005$), and hyperlipidemia ($p < 0.0005$), the correlation was $p < 0.0001$. With the
exception of stroke (rank 5), MAU ranked among the top four variables in all diseases, ranking as high as second for LVH and hypertensive retinopathy.

We also assessed the effects of treatment. The physicians did
not agree to a randomized trial, but instead wished to exercise their
prerogative in terms of assigning treatment. Thus, the patients were
treated with the monotherapy of the physicians' choice. The physicians were frequently asked to assign carvedilol, which was provided
free of charge by Boehringer Mannheim. Other choices included
beta-blockers, angiotensin-converting enzyme (ACE) inhibitors, calcium channel blockers, thiazide diuretics, and other agents, including
alpha-blocking drugs and centrally acting medications.

Demographic results, the effects on blood pressure by the antihypertensive regimens, and the effects on MAU at 3 months are shown in Table 3. The carvedilol group was about seven times larger than the ACE inhibitor and beta-blocker groups, and was much larger than the groups receiving only diuretic therapy or therapy with other drugs. The patients in the beta-blocker group were significantly younger by 6 or more years than those in the other groups. Height and weight were not different among the groups. The diuretic group and the group treated with other drugs contained somewhat more women than the other four groups. The duration of hypertension, the blood-pressure values, and the heart rate did not differ among the groups.

After 3 months of monotherapy, blood pressure had decreased by 20/12 mm Hg in the carvedilol group, 13/8 mm Hg in the ACE inhibitor group, 11/7 mm Hg in the beta-blocker group, 10/7 mm Hg in the calcium channel blocker group, 13/8 mm Hg in the diuretic group, and 9/6 mm Hg in the group treated with various other drugs. The blood-pressure decrease in the carvedilol group exceeded that in the other five groups ($p < 0.05$). Blood-pressure reductions in the other groups did not differ.

Also shown in Table 3 is the absolute number and the percentage of patients with MAU. These percentages were 38, 37, 24, 34, 32, and 26 in the groups assigned to the carvedilol, ACE inhibitor, beta-blocker, calcium channel blocker, diuretic, and other drug treatment groups, respectively. After 3 months of treatment, the numbers of MAU patients had decreased to 16%, 24%, 16%, 23%, 18%, and 21% in these treatment groups, respectively. Thus, the improvement rates (MAU patients who reverted to negative) in the carvedilol, ACE inhibitor, beta-blocker, calcium channel blocker, diuretic, and other drug group were 58%, 33%, 34%, 31%, 44%, and 20%, respectively. All blood-pressure-reducing therapies were successful in lowering the percentage of MAU patients.

We performed a stepwise linear-regression analysis on the patient population as a whole as well as on four of the treatment groups separately. The dependent variable in this analysis was reversal of MAU. For the entire population, decrease in systolic blood pressure, carvedilol treatment, decrease in diastolic blood pressure, heart rate,

Table 3 Demographic Results and Effects of Treatment on Blood Pressure and MAU in Mildly Hypertensive Patients Treated with Monotherapy

Group variable	CAR	ACE	BBL	CCB	DIU	Other
Number	4014	592	586	470	165	173
Age (years)	56±111	57±12	50±12*	60±11	60±13	60±13
Weight (kg)	79±13	79±14	79±14	78±12	76±13	78±13
Height (cm)	171±9	171±9	172±9	170±8	268±8	168±9
M/F (gender%)	52:48	56:44	54:46	53:47	41:59*	43:57*
Duration (months of hypertension)	56±60	64±66	56±59	67±66	70±68	75±76
Heart rate	77±9	77±9	77±11	78±9	80±10	78±10
Systolic (mm Hg)	168±17	164±18	159±17	162±18	161±18	161±19
Diastolic (mm Hg)	100±9	97±9	96±12	97±13	96±13	95±11
BP mm Hg (3 months)	148/88	150/89	147/89	151/89	147/88	152/89
Reduction (mm Hg)	20/12*	13/8	11/7	10/7	13/8	9/6
MAU (%)	38	37	24	34	32	26
MAU (%)(3 months)	16	24	16	23	18	21
MAU (% decrease)	58[a]	33	34	32	44	20

[a] $p < 0.05$ compared to other groups.
Mean ± SD.
CAR = carvedilol; ACE = angiotensin-converting enzyme inhibitors; BBL = beta-blockers; CCB = calcium channel blockers; DIU = diuretics; others = alpha-blockers and centrally acting agents.

duration of hypertension, height, and weight entered the analysis, in that order. For the carvedilol group, the decrease in diastolic blood pressure, duration of hypertension, decrease in systolic blood pressure, height, and weight entered the relationship. For ACE inhibitors and beta-blockers, the variable was the decrease in diastolic blood pressure. For calcium channel blockers, the variable was a reduction in systolic blood pressure. The numbers of subjects in the other groups were too small to allow for a meaningful analysis. With the application of an exponential rather than a linear fit, the same variables were associated with reversal of MAU from positive to negative in the entire population and within the various groups.

We surveyed a large hypertensive population receiving primary care in Germany. Ours cannot be considered a standardized prospective epidemiological investigation, since important standardization criteria, "blinded" blood-pressure determinations, and a randomized proband selection process were not included. These limitations should be considered when interpreting our findings. We observed that a qualitative estimate of MAU was strongly associated with complications in patients with essential hypertension. The prevalence of MAU in this hypertensive population of 11,343 patients was over 30%. Those with MAU were more likely to have coronary artery disease, LVH, stroke, and peripheral vascular disease. They had had hypertension for a longer time, were more likely to have lipid disturbances than hypertensive patients without MAU, had a greater degree of retinopathy, and had slight but significantly higher plasma creatinine values. Similarly, when the hypertensive complications were analyzed separately for MAU, patients with MAU were represented disproportionately compared to non-MAU patients in every instance. Finally, a stepwise multiple-regression analysis identified MAU as a risk factor independent of all other risk factors, such as age, duration of hypertension, and degree of blood-pressure elevation. These findings were not unexpected; each has been observed previously, albeit in much smaller numbers of patients. The contributions of this study are the size of the population and the facts that the patients were drawn from a general practice rather than from a referral population and that all the complications were monitored within the same population. We believe that this experience helps to establish the role of MAU as indicating cardiovascular risk in essential hypertension, and that it underscores the value of a simple and inexpensive screening method that can be performed in the physician's office or at home.

We used the Micral-Test to determine the presence of MAU (8). Semiquantitative methods have been criticized because of poor specificity, despite excellent sensitivity (9). The Micral-Test and another semiquantitative test were compared to four quantitative methods in which a double-antibody radioimmunoassay was used as the reference standard (10). In this comparison, the Micral-Test displayed a sensitivity of >90% and a specificity of 87%. Urine from our subjects was not examined by a quantitative method if positive. However, we feel that the large numbers of subjects in this study, coupled with the reasonable specificity of the Micral-Test, render our data reliable.

Our data confirmed the observation that MAU is associated with coronary artery disease and vascular disease elsewhere. Agrawal et al. (7) drew attention to MAU as a risk factor in nondiabetic hypertensive patients, and found that MAU predicted an outcome in these patients that is as dismal as that in patients with type II diabetes mellitus. Ljungman et al. (11) studied middle-aged hypertensive men with MAU, following them prospectively. One-third developed cardiovascular disease, much more than in a control group without MAU and similar blood pressures. The San Antonio Heart Study provided an opportunity to study this phenomenon further. Haffner et al. (12) found MAU in 42 (13%) of 316 nondiabetic Mexican Americans. These subjects had higher blood pressures, higher lipid values, higher insulin levels in response to glucose, and more myocardial infarctions than those who did not have MAU. MAU is associated not only with coronary artery disease, but also with LVH. Our data confirmed this observation as well. Redon et al. (13) first drew attention to this association. Pedrinelli et al. (14) confirmed these observations. Our patients with MAU were more likely to have peripheral vascular disease than those who did not. Patients with claudication appear prone to proteinuria. Hickey et al. (15) found that claudicants had a fivefold greater MAU excretion compared to controls; with exercise, this difference increased to 10-fold.

Our patients with MAU were more prone to exhibit hyperlipidemia and elevated creatinine values. Others have reported an association with MAU and high lipid values to varying degrees (16–18). Our MAU subjects had slightly higher creatinine values than non-MAU subjects. However, they were older, had had hypertension for a longer time, and had more vascular disease and more lipid disturbances. Abnormal increases in creatinine concentration (>1.8 mg/dl) were no more common in MAU than in non-MAU patients. Since overt proteinuria was an exclusion criterion, we did not expect to find significant numbers of patients with renal damage. Volhard and Fahr (19) were perhaps the first to draw attention to intermittent albuminuria in hypertensive patients, and suggested that poorly perfused, ischemic glomeruli might leak protein. The possibility that MAU might predict which individuals are at risk to develop hypertensive nephrosclerosis and renal failure has been raised by several authors (5,20,21) but not been confirmed by others (22–25).

CONCLUSIONS

The mechanisms of MAU in diabetic and hypertensive patients have received considerable attention. Endothelial damage seems to play a pertinent role. MAU is associated with smoking, which may injure the endothelium independent of other smoking-related effects (26). An important and regrettable omission was our failure to obtain smoking data on these patients. Von Willebrand's factor plasma concentrations have been found to be elevated in patients with type II diabetes mellitus and MAU (27). Von Willebrand's factor is produced by endothelial cells and contributes to the development of occlusive thrombosis (28). Its elevation in the plasma of persons with MAU supports the notion that MAU is indicative of ongoing endothelial damage.

We believe that our demonstrating the clinical utility of MAU in a practice setting has important implications. The semiquantitative test we used is not expensive and can be performed by a trained nurse or by the patients themselves (8–10). MAU determinations could have utility in selecting hypertensive patients requiring more detailed diagnostic approaches such as 24-hour blood-pressure monitoring (31,32), testing for salt sensitivity (33), echocardiography (13, 14), or vascular visualization (15). Moreover, MAU can be reduced by antihypertensive drugs (25). We suggest that qualitative MAU determinations in a practice setting would be of value in identifying high-risk patients and may play a role in their subsequent management.

Finally, our study shows that the treatment of hypertension with *any* medication reduces MAU in a practice setting. The present study was not a prospective, randomized, double-blind trial of antihypertensive agents and MAU. Instead, we performed a prospective open study of various monotherapies and their effect on MAU. Assignment of patients to treatment was neither random nor uniform. Thus, the carvedilol group was almost 10 times the size of all other groups, and more than 20 times larger than the diuretic group or the group containing patients treated with an alpha-blocker or centrally acting agents. Although we did not attempt to uniformly assign the patients, the groups were similar in terms of blood pressure, age, body size, duration of hypertension, and gender distribution. The carvedilol group contained a significantly larger proportion of MAU patients than the other groups. The physicians determined drug dosage at their discretion, although we asked the physicians to lower the blood pressures of their patients to within the normal range, or at least by 10 mm Hg in both systolic and diastolic blood pressures.

All antihypertensive treatments were successful in reducing MAU. Whether any single regimen among those tested was superior in terms of MAU reduction—or blood-pressure reduction, for that matter—cannot be determined from this nonrandomized, non-blinded study. We showed that the qualitative determination of MAU was precise in detecting high-risk nondiabetic hypertensive patients (7). However, to establish for certain that reversal of MAU indicates a reduction of cardiovascular risk in these patients would necessitate long-term prospective investigations. However, the qualitative test for MAU is not expensive and requires no laboratory or extra medical personnel. Our data show that reversal of MAU during drug treatment can readily be determined. We suggest that MAU, if present, should be measured and monitored in nondiabetic hypertensive patients. Reduced MAU should be a therapeutic goal.

REFERENCES

1. Viberti GC, Hill RD, Jarrett RJ. Microalbuminuria as a predictor of clinical nephropathy in insulin-dependent diabetes mellitus. Lancet 1982; i:1430–1432.
2. Neil A, Thorogood M, Hawkins M, Cohen D, Potok M, Mann J. A prospective population-based study of microalbuminuria as a predictor of mortality in NIDDM. Diabetes Care 1993; 16:996–1003.
3. Mimran A, Ribstein J. Microalbuminuria in essential hypertension. Clin Exp Hypertens 1993; 15:1061–1067.
4. Ljungman S. Microalbuminuria in essential hypertension. Am J Hypertens 1990; 3(12 Pt 1):956–960.

5. Rambausek M, Fliser D, Ritz E. Albuminuria of hypertensive patients. Clin Nephrol 1992; 38(suppl 1):S40–S45.
6. Ritz E, Fliser D. Clinical relevance of albuminuria in hypertensive patients. Clin Investig 1992; 70(suppl 1):5114–5119.
7. Agrawal B, Berger A, Wolf K, Luft FC. Microalbumin screening by reagent strip predicts cardiovascular risk in hypertension. J Hypertens 1996. In press.
8. Marshall SM, Shearing PA, Alberti KGMM. Micral-Test strips evaluated for screening for albuminuria. Clin Chem 1992; 38:588–591.
9. Biampietro O, Penno G, Clerico A, Cruschelli L, Lucchetti A, Nannipieri M, Cecere M, Rizzo L, Navalesi R. Which method for quantifying "microalbuminuria" in diabetics?: comparison of several immunological methods for measurement of albumin in urine. Acta Diabetol 1992; 28:239–245.
10. Tiu SC, Lee SS, Cheng MW. Comparison of six commercial techniques in the measurement of microalbuminuria in diabetic patients. Diabetes Care 1993; 16:616–620.
11. Ljungman S, Auurell M, Hartford M. Blood pressure and renal function. Acta Med Scand 1980; 208:17–25.
12. Haffner SM, Stern MP, Gruber MK, Hazuda HP, Mitchell BD, Patterson JK. Microalbuminuria: potential marker for increased cardiovascular risk factors in nondiabetic subjects? Arteriosclerosis 1990; 10: 727–731.
13. Redon J, Gomez-Sanchez MA, Baldo E, Casal MC, Fermandez M, Miralles A, Gomez-Pajuelo C, Rodicio JL, Ruilope LM. Micro-albuminuria is correlated with left ventricular hypertrophy in male hypertensive patients. J Hypertens 1991; 9(suppl 6):5148–5149.
14. Pedrinelli R, Di Bello V, Catapano G, Talarico L, Materazzi F, Santoro G, Giusti C, Mosca F, Melillo E, Ferrari M. Microalbuminuria is a marker of left ventricular hypertrophy but not hyperinsulemia in nondiabetic atherosclerotic patients. Arterioscler Thromb 1993; 13:900–906.
15. Hickey NC, Shearman CP, Gosling P, Simms MH. Assessment of intermittent claudication by quantitation of exercise-induced microalbuminuria. Eur J Vasc Surg 1990; 4:603–606.
16. Niskanen L, Uusitupa M, Sarlund H, Siitonen O, Voutilainen E, Penttilae I, Pyoeraelae K. Microalbuminuria predicts the development of serum lipoprotein abnormalities favoring atherogenesis in newly diagnosed type 2 (non-insulin-dependent) diabetic patients. Diabetologia 1990; 33:237–243.

17. Reverter JL, Santi M, Rubies-Prat J, Lucas A, Salinas I, Pizzaro E, Pedro-Botet J, Romero R, Sanmarti A. Relationship between lipoprotein profile and urinary albumin excretion in type II diabetic patients with stable metabolic control. Diabetes Care 1994; 17:189–194.
18. Smellie WSA, Warwick GL. Primary hyperlipidemia is not associated with increased urinary albumin excretion. Nephrol Dialysis Transpl 1991; 6:398–401.
19. Volhard F, Fahr T. Die Bright'sche Nierenkrankheit. Klinik, Pathologie und Atlas. Berlin: Springer, 1914:225.
20. Kaplan NM. Microalbuminuria: a risk factor for vascular and renal complications of hypertension. Am J Med 1992; 92(48):8S–12S.
21. Cerasola G, Cottone S, D'Ignoto G. Microalbuminuria points out early renal and cardiovascular changes in essential hypertension. Rev Lat Cardiol 1992; 13:3–7.
22. Bigazzi R, Bianchi S, Campese V, Baldari G. Prevalence of microalbuminuria in a large population of patients with mild to moderate essential hypertension. Nephron 1992; 61:94–97.
23. Ljungman S, Wikstrand J, Hartford M, Aurell M, Lindstedt G, Berglund G. Effects of long-term antihypertensive treatment and aging on renal function and albumin excretion in primary hypertension. Am J Hypertens 1993; 6:554–563.
24. Lindeman RD, Tobin JD, Shock NW. Association between blood pressure and the rate of decline in renal function with age. Kidney Int 1984; 26:861–868.
25. Ruilope LM, Alcazar JM, Hernandez E, Praga M, Lahera V, Rodicio JL. Long-term influences of antihypertensive therapy on microalbuminuria in essential hypertension. Kidney Int 1994; 45(suppl):5171–5173.
26. Corradi L, Zoppi A, Tettamanti F, Malamani GD, Lazzari P, Fogari R. Smoking habits and microalbuminuria in hypertensive patients with type 2 diabetes mellitus. J Hypertens 1993; 11:S190–S191.
27. Stehouwer CD, Nauta JJ, Yeldenrust GC, Hackeng WH, Donker AJ. Urinary albumin excretion, cardiovascular disease, and endothelial dysfunction in non-insulin-dependent diabetes mellitus. Lancet 1992; 340: 319–323.
28. Nichols TC, Bellinger DA, Tate DA. Von Willebrand factor and occlusive arterial thrombosis: a study in normal and Von Willebrand's disease pigs with diet induced hypercholesterolemia and atherosclerosis. Arterioscler Thromb 1990; 10:449–461.
29. Pedrinelli R, Giampietro O, Carmassi F, Melillo E, Dell'Oma G, Catapano G, Matteucci E, Talarico L, Morale M, De Negri F, Di Bello V.

Microalbuminuria and endothelial dysfunction in essential hypertension. Lancet 1994; 344:14–18.

30. Grunden G, Cavallo-Perin P, Bazzan M, Stella S, Vuolo A, Pagano G.
PAI-1 and factor VII activity are higher in IDDM patients with microalbuminuria. Diabetes 1994; 43:426–429.

31. Giaconi S, Levanti C, Fommei E, Innocenti F, Segheri G, Palla L,
Palombo C, Ghione S. Microalbuminuria and casual and ambulatory
blood pressure monitoring in normotensives and in patients with borderline and mild essential hypertension. Am J Hypertens 1989; 2:259–
261.

32. Bianchi S, Bigazzi R, Baldari G, Sgherri G, Campese VM. Diurnal vari-
ations of blood pressure and microalbuminuria in essential hypertension. Am J Hypertens 1994; 7:23–29.

33. Bigazzi R, Bianchi S, Baldari D, Sgherri G, Baldari G, Campese VM.
Microalbuminuria in salt-sensitive patients: a marker for renal and cardiovascular risk factors. Hypertension 1994; 23:195–199.

9

Improvement of Coronary Microcirculation by ACE Inhibitors

S. Scheler and W. Motz   Ernst-Moritz-Arndt-Universität Greifswald, Greifswald, Germany

B. E. Strauer   Heinrich-Heine-Universität Düsseldorf, Düsseldorf, Germany

Disturbance of coronary microcirculation is most frequently caused by arterial hypertension. Even if their epicardial coronary arteries are normal, patients with arterial hypertension often have symptoms of angina pectoris and a positive exercise tolerance test. The symptoms of angina pectoris in patients with arterial hypertension are due to functional and structural alterations of the coronary microcirculation. Consequently, antihypertensive therapy should aim not only at lowering blood pressure and reversing myocardial hypertrophy, but also at improving coronary microcirculation to avoid the effects of chronic ischemia on the myocardium.

Until now, the studies indicating that antihypertensive therapy can improve coronary flow reserve have been experimental. To determine whether coronary flow reserve can be improved in hypertensives under clinical conditions, maximal coronary blood flow, minimal coronary resistance, and coronary reserve (dipyridamole) were studied before and after long-term antihypertensive treatment (9–12 months) with the ACE inhibitor enalapril (10–20 mg/day). To assess the chronic rather than the acute effects of the antihypertensive pharmacon, coronary microcirculation was studied after intermission of medical therapy for a period of 1 week. Along with a decrease in left ventricular muscle mass by about 8%, coronary reserve was improved after enalapril by 48%. It is likely that the observed increase in coronary reserve is related to the reversal of structural vascular abnormalities on the level of the coronary microcirculation. Consequently, it seems that reparation of hypertensive remodeling of the coronary microcirculation can be induced by ACE-inhibitor therapy.

INTRODUCTION

Left ventricular hypertrophy is a serious risk factor of cardiovascular complications such as myocardial infarction, stroke, and congestive heart failure (1). In contrast to adaptive myocardial hypertrophy due to athletic training, LV hypertrophy due to arterial hypertension is characterized by growth or altered metabolism of nonmyocytic cells such as cardiac fibroblasts, smooth-muscle cells, and endothelial cells (2). These functional and structural activations of nonmyocytic cells greatly alter the myocardial structure function. Since an activation of nonmyocytic cells can be also present without a concomitant myocardial hypertrophy, its activation is not inevitably linked to the myocytic hypertrophy process.

Consequently, a causative therapy of hypertensive hypertrophy must aim at a specific reparation of the organ structure of heart and circulation. This can be realized through a specific intervention on the level of the nonmyocytic cells such as cardiofibroblasts in the interstitial space, vascular smooth-muscle cells, and endothelial cells. A therapeutic intervention on the level of only the myocytes leads to echocardiographic regression of myocardial hypertrophy, and the decisive reparation of the remodeled organ structure may thus fail to occur. Accordingly, the aim of interventional therapy of the heart in hypertension is not merely the echocardiographic decrement of

REPAIR OF HYPERTENSIVE CARDIAC REMODELING

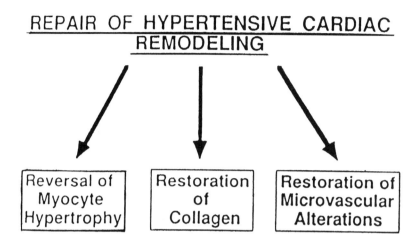

Figure 1   Concept of cardioreparation of hypertensive remodeling.

wall thickness, i.e., reversal of hypertrophy, but the basic reparation of the myocardial structure remodeled by hypertension. This particularly comprises the myocardial interstitial space, i.e., connective tissue and the coronary microcirculation (2) (Figure 1).

STUDIES

Patients with arterial hypertension often have symptoms of angina pectoris even with a normal coronary angiogram (3–5). About 50% of the hypertensive patients with a normal coronary angiogram who were admitted to the Department of Cardiology of the University of Düsseldorf because of clinically suspected coronary artery disease had typical exercise-related and nitroglycerine-responsive angina. Of these patients, 42% showed clearly pathological exercise-tolerance test results in spite of having smooth epicardial arteries. Consequently, a normal coronary angiogram does not exclude alterations of the coronary circulation. Small coronary arterioles and resistance vessels with a diameter of less than 150 μm of the coronary microcirculation are beyond the resolution of coronary angiography. A normal coronary angiogram indicates only the absence of visible alterations of the great epicardial conductance arteries.

In patients with arterial hypertension, maximal coronary blood flow due to dipyridamole is lowered by about 35% compared with healthy normotensive control persons. Accordingly, minimal coronary resistance as the reciprocal parameter of coronary conductance is appropriately elevated, and coronary reserve, defined as the quotient of coronary resistance under resting conditions and minimal coronary resistance after dipyridamole, is lowered by about 30% (5–7). Consequently, patients with arterial hypertension and angina pectoris frequently show functional impairment of the coronary regulation capacity on the level of the coronary microcirculation. Possible causes of the disturbed coronary flow reserve in arterial hypertension are of vascular, myocardial, and metabolic origin. Tomanek et al. (8) described rarefaction of the coronary microcirculation as the consequence of inadequate growth of the capillaries along with the process of hypertrophy in experimental models of arterial hypertension. Furthermore, in experimental studies a thickening of the walls of resistance arteries in the form of medial hypertrophy was found (9). Such findings could also be observed in myocardial biopsies of patients in arterial hypertension (10). Further, perivascular fibrosis as well as a disturbance of coronary endothelial function, meaning a reduced capacity of EDRF liberation, have been discussed as being causative for the impaired flow reserve (11,12).

Besides these vascular factors, myocardial hypertrophy remains a main determinant of the extravascular component of the coronary resistance as another reason for the impaired coronary flow reserve. Qualitative alterations of myocardial structure in the sense of interstitial fibrosis might have an unfavorable impact on coronary microcirculation. In particular, diastolic compression of the endocardial areas of the myocardium through the elevated LV filling pressure might contribute to the impairment of coronary regulatory capacity as well. Due to an elevated instantaneous coronary flow as a consequence of an elevated myocardial energy demand, coronary reserve can be metabolically impaired in the absence of microvascular alterations. Such a metabolically caused limitation of coronary flow reserve is found particularly in hemodynamically decompensated left ventricles due to prolonged exposure to arterial hypertension and in patients with aortic valve disease (3,13).

The structural remodeling of the myocardium along with the process of arterial hypertension is not caused solely by the physical pressure load on the cardiac myocytes, but also by the interrelationship of mechanical stretch, i.e., systolic wall stretch and hormonal stimulation. Besides adrenergic stimulation (14–16), the renin-angiotensin system particularly modulates the hypertrophy process of myocytes and smooth-muscle cells and induces proto-oncogenes, which induce or reinforce the process of hypertrophy. The development of LV hypertrophy due to coarctation of the abdominal aorta in rats could be completely prevented after pretreatment with an ACE inhibitor (17). This speaks in favor of a decisive tropic role of angiotensin II on the myocardium and the antitropic effect of the therapeutic inhibition of the renin-angiotensin system.

During the process of adaptive myocardial hypertrophy due to arterial hypertension, the cardiac endogenous ACE activity as well as messenger RNA of ACE is elevated. Schunkert and coworkers (18) have found a rise in ACE mRNA and an increased conversion of angiotensin I to angiotensin II in the pressure-exposed left ventricle. In the non-pressure-exposed right ventricle, ACE activity was not different from that in control animals. Consequently, the stimulus of increased ACE expression is locally linked to the muscle fiber stretch as a consequence of the increased systolic wall stress in the pressure-loaded left ventricle. The evidence of induction of proto-oncogenes through angiotensin II supports the assumption that hypertensive remodeling of the heart is modulated through the local and endocrine renin-angiotensin system (19,20).

Given the importance of the renin-angiotensin system in the process of hypertensive remodeling of the heart and circulation, ACE inhibitors are an obvious choice in medical treatment of arterial hypertension. Many experimental and clinical studies (21–24) have clearly shown that therapy with ACE inhibitors induces regression of myocardial hypertrophy (Figure 2). At least experimentally, in the spontaneously hypertensive rat, Brilla and coworkers (25) have found a reversal of the interstitial collagen as well as a decrement of

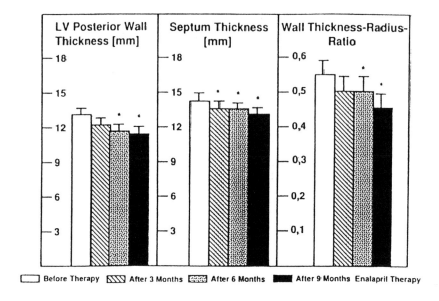

Figure 2 Left ventricular posterior wall thickness, septum thickness, and ratio of wall thickness to radius before and 3, 6, and 9 months after therapy with enalapril. *$p < 0.05$.

the medial wall thickness of coronary resistance vessels after long-term treatment with the ACE inhibitor lisinopril. Functionally, an improvement of the coronary flow reserve was found in the lisinopril-treated animals. A decrement of the vascular wall thickness of the large peripheral conductance arteries was found after antihypertensive therapy with the ACE inhibitors enalapril and perindopril in the same experimental model of hypertension. These latter findings were interpreted as reflecting an antiproliferative effect of ACE inhibitors on vascular smooth-muscle cells (26,27).

Until now it has not been clear whether clinical antihypertensive therapy with an ACE inhibitor can also improve or even normalize the obvious disturbance of coronary microcirculation in arterial hypertension. To answer this question, we studied patients with hypertensive microvascular angina pectoris, i.e.: a) a history of arterial hypertension, b) symptoms of angina pectoris and/or c) evidence of myocardial ischemia in the exercise-tolerance test or thallium scan, d) normal epicardial arteries, and e) an impaired coronary flow reserve. As a antihypertensive treatment we chose the ACE inhibitor enalapril because of its likely antiproliferative effects on the vasculature. After discontinuation of a preexisting antihypertensive therapy for 1 week, coronary circulation and LV muscle mass were studied. After that, the patients were treated with enalapril (10–20 mg/day) for 9 to 12 months. To assess the chronic effect of antihypertensive treatment on coronary microcirculation rather than the acute effect of enalapril, coronary circulation was studied after the medical therapy had been discontinued for a period of 1 week. The objective of the study was to assess the chronic effect of long-term antihypertensive treatment with enalapril on the coronary microcirculation and not the acute effect of the antihypertensive substance (28,29).

During antihypertensive treatment with enalapril, systolic and diastolic blood-pressure values were within the normotensive range. The reduction of systolic blood pressure was about 20 mm Hg and the reduction of the diastolic blood pressure about 8–10 mm Hg. LV muscle mass decreased from 268 $\pm$ 58 g to 247 $\pm$ 50 g ($p < 0.05$). It is notable that in all patients no marked LV hypertrophy existed initially (28,29).

Before and after discontinuation of enalapril therapy, coronary perfusion pressure, heart rate, myocardial oxygen consumption, and pulmonary capillary wedge pressure were similar. Consequently, measurement of coronary regulatory capacity was measured under identical perfusion pressures before and after therapy, and there were also no obvious differences with respect to myocardial energy consumption and heart rate as well as in the end-diastolic compressing forces under both conditions. After the treatment period, maximal coronary blood flow after dipyridamole increased by 43%, from 181 $\pm$ 69 to 258 $\pm$ 116 ml/min·100 g ($p < 0.001$). Minimal coronary resistance as the reciprocal parameter of coronary conductance decreased by 29%, from 0.66 $\pm$ 0.23 to 0.47 $\pm$ 0.24 mm Hg/min·100 g/ml ($p < 0.001$). Coronary reserve was improved by 48% compared with its initial value (28,29) (Figure 3).

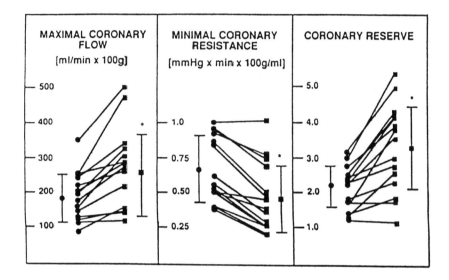

Figure 3 Effects of long-term treatment with enalapril on coronary vaso-
dilating capacity. A significant increase in maximal coronary flow and decrease in minimal coronary resistance occurred in response to dipyridamole
(0.5 mg/kg body weight i.v.), with a corresponding increase in coronary reserve. Minimal coronary resistance did not change in only one patient.

Since coronary reserve has improved chronically—i.e., independently from the acute effect of the antihypertensive agent—regression of structural alterations on the level of the myocardium and
the coronary resistance vessels is likely to have occurred. For example, a decrease in medial wall thickness and in perivascular fibrosis,
as well as an increase in capillary density, are possible. On the myocardial level, a decrease in myocytic hypertrophy and a possible decrease in the amount of the interstitial collagen concentration must
be considered. Until now, the influence of chronic medical therapy
on coronary microcirculation has been studied experimentally only
in the model of the spontaneously hypertensive rat. Anderson and
coworkers (30) found an increase in coronary flow reserve without a
concomitant reversal of myocardial hypertrophy along with chronic
antihypertensive treatment with hydralazine. From this study it was

concluded that alteration of the myocardial factor is not a prerequisite for improvement of coronary flow reserve.

Strauer (4) showed that chronic therapy with the calcium channel blocker felodipin led to a decrement in medial wall thickness along with an increase in coronary flow reserve. Others (31–33) found an increase in the capillary density of the myocardium after chronic therapy with nifedipine, moxonidine, and captopril. Mall and coworkers (32) found, in addition to an increase in capillary density, a decrement in LV muscle mass of the left ventricle and a decrease in medial wall thickness after nifedipine and moxonidine.

An increase in coronary regulatory capacity was observed following treatment with the ACE inhibitors captopril (31) and lisinopril (25). Canby and Tomanek (31) attributed the increase in coronary regulatory capacity to the increase in capillary density, and Brilla and coworkers (25) to both reversal of LV muscle mass and a decrease in medial wall thickness of the coronary resistance arteries.

In conclusion, these experimental studies have demonstrated that chronic therapy with various antihypertensive drugs will lead to reversal of myocytic hypertrophy on the level of the myocardium as well as to a decrease in medial wall thickness and an increase in the capillary density on the level of the coronary microcirculation. Functionally, the coronary regulatory capacity of the coronary microcirculation increases.

Through the concomitant reversal of hypertrophy along with blood-pressure reduction, a decrease of the myocardial component of the coronary resistance inevitably occurs. Consequently, it is difficult to differentiate between the influence on the coronary flow reserve of the myocardial factors, such as hypertrophy and fibrosis, and the vascular factors, such as medial wall thickening and capillary density, under experimental as well as clinical conditions. Under clinical conditions, a distinct decrease (29%) in minimal coronary resistance as the reciprocal parameter of coronary conductance occurred along with a moderate amount of reversal of myocardial hypertrophy due to enalapril treatment (28,29). In contrast, in spite of a distinct reversal of myocardial hypertrophy, an insignificant decrease (11%) in minimal coronary resistance was found after chronic treatment with the beta-receptor-blocker bisoprolol (28,34).

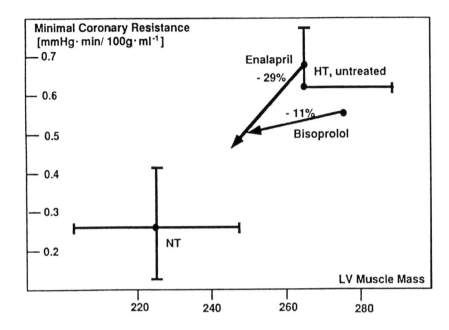

Figure 4 (Abscissa) Left ventricular muscle mass and (ordinate) minimal coronary resistance. In normotensive control persons, a normal minimal coronary resistance exists in the presence of a normal LV muscle mass. In hypertensive patients, minimal coronary vascular resistance is significantly increased along with the presence of LV hypertrophy. After therapy with enalapril (left arrow), a distinct decrease in minimal coronary resistance occurs in spite of an only moderate decrease in myocardial hypertrophy. Under treatment with the beta-receptor-blocker bisoprolol (right arrow), a moderate insignificant decrease in minimal coronary resistance occurs in spite of clear reversal of myocardial hypertrophy. Consequently, a) an influence on the myocardial factor "left ventricular hypertrophy" does not automatically lead to an improvement of conductance of the coronary microcirculation and b) an improvement of coronary conductance after enalapril cannot be the sole consequence of reversal of hypertrophy. Accordingly, additional vascular effects of the enalapril treatment seem to be responsible for the improvement in coronary flow reserve.

These findings demonstrate that a sole influence on the myocardial factor LV hypertrophy does not necessarily lead to a distinct improvement of conductance of the coronary microcirculation, and that improvement of coronary conductance due to enalapril therapy cannot be caused only by regression of myocardial hypertrophy. Furthermore, additional vascular effects of the ACE inhibitor enalapril are likely (Figure 4). This interpretation is supported by experimental findings of Christensen and coworkers (35). They demonstrated that the media-lumen ratio of mesenteric resistance arteries was distinctly lower after treatment with the vasodilators captopril, hydralazine, and isradipine than after the beta-receptor-blocker metoprolol.

The only study on human coronary resistance vessels was published by Heagerty and coworkers (36). They found a plane decrement of the ratio between medial wall thickness and lumen diameter in subcutaneous resistance vessels after antihypertensive combination therapy. Based on these studies of the peripheral circulation (35,36) and the experimental studies (25–27) that have shown an antiproliferative effect of ACE inhibitors on the vessel wall, it is likely that the improved coronary flow reserve with enalapril is caused by reparation of structural vascular alterations of the coronary microcirculation, such as a decrease in medial wall thickness and perivascular fibrosis. Furthermore, a quantitative decrement in interstitial myocardial fibrosis might also have contributed in the form of a decrement in the myocardial component of coronary resistance.

CONCLUSION

Chronic therapy with the ACE inhibitor enalapril must be considered a cardioreparative treatment. It restores the structural integrity in hypertensive heart disease because reversal of myocytic hypertrophy, a decrease in myocardial fibrosis, and a near-normalization of the coronary microcirculation can be realized.

REFERENCES

1. Levy D, Garrison RJ, Savage DD, Kannel WB, Castelli WP. Prognostic implications of echocardiographically determined left ventricular mass in the Framingham Heart Study. N Engl J Med 1990; 322:1561–1566.

2. Weber KT, Anversa P, Armstrong PW, Brilla CG, Burnett JC, Crnick-shank JM, Devereux RB, Giles TD, Korsgaard N, Leier CV, Mendel-sohn FAO, Motz WH, Mulvany MJ, Strauer BE. Remodeling and reparation of the cardiovascular system. J Am Coll Cardiol 1992; 20: 3–16.
3. Strauer BE. Myocardial oxygen consumption in chronic heart disease: role of wall stress, hypertrophy and coronary reserve. Am J Cardiol 1979; 44:730–740.
4. Strauer BE. The significance of coronary reserve in clinical heart disease. J Am Coll Cardiol 1990; 15:775–783.
5. Strauer BE. Hypertensive Heart Disease. Berlin: Springer, 1983.
6. Motz W, Vogt M, Scheler S, Schwartzkopff, B, Strauer BE. Coronary circulation in arterial hypertension. J Cardiovasc Pharmacol 1991; 17 (suppl 23):S35–S39.
7. Vogt M, Motz W, Strauer BE. Coronary flow reserve in arterial hypertension. Scand J Clin Lab Invest 1989; 49(suppl 196):7–15.
8. Tomanek RJ, Palmer PJ, Pfeiffer GL, Schreiber KL, Eastham GL, Marcus ML. Morphometry of canine coronary arteries, arterioles and capillaries during hypertension and left ventricular hypertrophy. Circ Res 1986; 58:38–46.
9. Plunkett WG, Overbeck HW. Arteriolar wall thickening in hypertensive rats unrelated to pressure or sympathoadrenergic influences. Circ Res 1988; 63:937–943.
10. Schwartzkopff B, Motz W, Knauer S, Frenzel H, Strauer BE. Morphometrische Untersuchung intramyokardialer Arteriolen aus Endomyokardbiopsien des rechtsventrikulären Septums bei Patienten mit arterieller Hypertonie und Linksherzhypertrophie. In: Ganten D, Mall G, Hrsg. Gefäß- und Herzhypertrophie. Stuttgart: Schattauer, 1992: 33–43.
11. Lüscher TF, Raij L, Vanhoutte PM. Endothelium-dependent vascular responses in normotensive and hypertensive Dahl rats. Hypertension 1987; 9:157–163.
12. Motz W, Vogt M, Rabenau O, Scheler S, Lückhoff A, Strauer BE. Evidence of endothelial dysfunction in coronary resistance vessels in patients with angina pectoris and normal coronary angiograms. Am J Cardiol 1991; 68:996–1003.
13. Eberli FR, Ritter M, Schwitter J, Bortone A, Schneider J, Hess OM, Krayenbühl HP. Coronary reserve in patients with aortic valve disease before and after successful aortic valve replacement. Eur Heart J 1991; 12:127–138.
14. Laks MMN. Norepinephrine—the myocardial hypertrophy hormone? Am Heart J 1976; 91:674–675.

15. Östman-Smith I. Cardiac sympathetic nerves as the final common pathway in the induction of adaptive cardiac hypertrophy. Clin Sci 1981; 61: 265–272.
16. Tarazi RC, Sen S, Saragoca M, Kairallah P. The multifactorial role of catecholamines in hypertensive cardiac hypertrophy. Eur Heart J 1982; suppl 3:A103–A110.
17. Kromer EP, Riegger GAJ. Effects of long-term angiotensin converting enzyme inhibition on myocardial hypertrophy in experimental aortic stenosis in the rat. Am J Cardiol 1988; 62:161–163.
18. Schunkert H, Dzau VJ, Tang SS, Hirsch AT, Apstein CS, Corell BH. Increased rat cardiac angiotensin converting enzyme activity and mRNA expression in pressure overload left ventricular hypertrophy. J Clin Invest 1990; 86:1913–1920.
19. Naftilan AJ, Pratt RE, Eldrige CS, Lin HL, Dzau VJ. Angiotensin II induces c-fos expression in smooth muscle via transcriptional control. Hypertension 1989; 13:706–711.
20. Naftilan AJ, Pratt RE, Dzau VJ. Induction of platelet-derived growth factor A chain and c-myc gene expressions by angiotensin II in cultured rat vascular smooth muscle cells. J Clin Invest 1989; 83:1419–1424.
21. Cruickshank JM. Reversibility of left ventricular hypertrophy (LVH) by differing types of antihypertensive therapy. J Hum Hypertens 1992; 6:85–90.
22. Motz W, Strauer BE. Rückbildung der hypertensiven Herzhypertrophie durch chronische Angiotensin-Konversionsenzymhemmung. Z Kardiol 1988; 77:53–60.
23. Nakashima Y, Fouad FM, Tarazi RC. Regression of left ventricular hypertrophy from systemic hypertension by enalapril. Am J Cardiol 1984; 53:1044–1049.
24. Sen S, Tarazi RC, Bumpus FM. Reversal of cardiac hypertrophy in renal hypertensive rats: medical vs. surgical therapy. Am J Physiol 1981; 270:H408–412.
25. Brilla CG, Janicki JS, Weber KT. Cardioreparative effects of lisinopril in rats with genetic hypertension and left ventricular hypertrophy. Circulation 1991; 83:1771–1779.
26. Clozel JP, Kuhn H, Hefti F. Effects of chronic ACE inhibition on cardiac hypertrophy and coronary vascular reserve in spontaneously hypertensive rats with developed hypertension. J Hypertens 1989; 7:267–275.
27. Michel JB, Levy BI. Vascular effects of ACE inhibition by pereindopril. Drugs 1990; 39(suppl 1):39–42.

28. Motz W, Vogt M, Scheler S, Schwartzkopff BE, Kelm M, Strauer BE. Prophylaxe mit gefäßakitiven Substanzen. Z Kardiol 1992; 81(suppl 4): 199–204.
29. Motz W, Strauer BE. Improvement of coronary reserve by chronic treatment: long-term therapy with enalapril. Hypertension 1996; 27:1031–1038.
30. Anderson PG, Bishop SP, Digerness SB. Vascular remodeling and improvement of coronary reserve after hydralazine treatment in spontaneously hypertensive rats. Circ Res 1989; 64:1127–1136.
31. Canby CA, Tomanek RJ. Role of lowering arterial pressure on maximal coronary flow with and without regression of cardiac hypertrophy. Am J Physiol 1989; 257 (Heart Circ Physiol 26):H1110–H1118.
32. Mall G, Greber D, Gharebhagi H, Wiest G, Mattfeldt T, Ganten U. Myokardprotektion und Hypertrophieregression bei spontan hypertensiven Ratten durch Nifedipin und Moxonidin. Stereologische Untersuchungen. In: Ganten D, Mall G, eds. Hrsg. Herz-Kreislauf-Regulation, Organprotektion und Organscheden. Stuttgart: Schattauer, 1991: 91–106.
33. Turek Z, Kubat K, Kazda S, Hoofd V, Rahnsan K. Improved myocardial capillarisation in spontaneously hypertensive rats treated with nifedipine. Cardiovasc Res 1987; 21:725–729.
34. Motz W, Vogt M, Scheler S, Schwartzkopff B, Strauer BE. Verbesserung der Koronarreserve nach Hypertrophieregression durch antihypertensive Therapie mit einem Beta-Rezeptorenblocker. Dt Med Wochenschr 1993; 118:535–540.
35. Christensen KL, Jespersen LT, Mulvany MJ. Development of blood pressure in spontaneously hypertensive rats after withdrawal of long-term treatment related to resistance vessel structure. J Hypertens 1989; 7:83–90.
36. Heagerty AM, Bund SJ, Aalkjaer C. Effects of drug treatment on human resistance ateriole morphology in essential hypertension: direct evidence for structural remodelling of resistance vessels. Lancet 1988; 1209–1212.

10

Dialysis Regimens and Myocardial Hypertrophy

W. H. M. van Kuijk and K. M. L. Leunissen   University Hospital Maastricht, Maastricht, The Netherlands

A. J. Luik   St. Maartens Gasthuis, Venlo, The Netherlands

INTRODUCTION

Cardiac disease is a major cause of death in patients with end-stage renal disease (ESRD). According to the European registry, cardiovascular causes account for 50% or more of deaths in both hemodialysis and continuous ambulatory peritoneal dialysis (CAPD) patients (1). With respect to cardiovascular disease, left ventricular hypertrophy (LVH) has been shown to be the most predominant structural finding in patients with ESRD. In a cross-sectional study, Harnett et al. (2) found an incidence of LVH (LV wall thickness ≥ 1.2 cm in diastole) of 65% in nondiabetic patients treated with hemodialysis. In a large multicenter prospective study, Foley et al. (3) reported an incidence of LVH (mass index >100 g/m2 in females and >131 g/m2 in males) of 74% in patients starting with ESRD therapy, including diabetics. At baseline, only 15.5% had a completely normal echo-cardiogram.

Generally, LVH progresses with time. Parfrey et al. (4) found that in a group of patients with either a normal echocardiogram or mild LVH, 16% progressed to severe LVH during a follow-up period of 3–5 years. Hüting et al. (5) found a significant increase only in the interventricular septum diameter while muscle mass remained unchanged, studying 61 normotensive dialysis patients during a follow-up period of 2.5 years.

LVH has been shown to be an important independent determinant of survival in dialysis patients (6). The cumulative survival was found to be significantly lower (53%) in patients with severe LVH than in patients with a normal echocardiogram (97%) or patients with mild LVH (85%) (4). LVH is associated with an increased risk of premature ventricular contractions, cardiac arrhythmias, and sudden death (7).

Thus, LVH is a frequent finding in patients with ESRD, and clearly influences patient survival negatively. Since LVH progresses in patients on ESRD therapy, the question arises of whether a specific interaction exists between the dialysis treatment itself and LVH. Conversely, LVH could have important implications for intradialytic hemodynamics.

ETIOLOGY

Three forms of LVH are recognized: concentric hypertrophy, asymmetrical septal hypertrophy, and eccentric or dilated hypertrophy. Concentric hypertrophy consists of an overall increase in wall thickness while the ventricular volume remains unchanged, resulting in an elevated mass/volume ratio. Asymmetrical septum hypertrophy consists of a predominant hypertrophy of the interventricular septum. Both forms are related to an increase in systolic stress due to chronic pressure overload or a decrease in aortic compliance (volume–pressure relationship). They are associated with diastolic dysfunction while systolic function remains normal or is even supernormal. In eccentric hypertrophy, both the left ventricular mass and volume are increased. The mass/volume ratio remains unchanged. This form of LVH has been related to chronic volume or flow overload (hyperdynamic state) as a result of anemia, hypervolemia, or the arteriovenous fistula. Dilated LVH is associated with systolic dysfunction as a result of an inadequate increase in ventricular mass for the degree of dilatation (4,5,8,9).

LVH has also been related to the uremic state itself. Experimental uremia in rats resulted in a significant increase in total heart weight as a result of an increase in volume density of interstitial tissue with ultimate deposition of collagen. This phenomenon could be dissociated from sympathetic overactivity, hypertension, and a hyperdynamic state due to hypervolemia (10–12). A diffuse interstitial fibrosis has also been found in the hearts of uremic patients (13). Parathyroid hormone might be recognized as a specific uremic toxin in relation to LVH. London et al. (14) found a correlation between the severity of the increase in the ratio of left ventricular radius to wall thickness and both serum PTH level and bone histological signs of osteitis fibrosa. Also, a decrease in left ventricular mass has been reported after parathyroidectomy (15).

In epidemiological studies, LVH has also been related to hemodynamic factors, anemia, and hyperparathyroidism. Harnett et al. (2) analyzed a group of 103 nondiabetic patients treated with either hemodialysis or CAPD, of which 68% had LVH. In this group, only age was identified as a significant risk factor for LVH although systolic blood pressure was significantly higher in the group with LVH than in those without LVH. A high level of serum alkaline phosphatase was the best predictor for severe LVH. Greaves et al. (16) evaluated potential risk factors for LVH in 38 undialysed patients with chronic renal failure, 54 patients treated with CAPD, and 30 patients treated with hemodialysis, including diabetics. In their study, LVH was positively correlated with systolic and diastolic blood pressures and inversely correlated with hematocrit. They could not find a relationship between LVH and secondary hyperparathyroidism. In a prospective study, Harnett et al. (17) followed a cohort of 51 dialysis patients who were free of LVH at the start of dialysis therapy. Development of LVH was associated with increased systolic blood pressure and older age.

DIALYSIS REGIMENS

Intradialytic Hemodynamics

Maintenance of cardiac output by adequate cardiac filling plays a key role in the regulation of blood pressure when blood volume declines as a result of ultrafiltration. However, when ventricular compliance is decreased in the presence of LVH, higher filling pressures are necessary to maintain cardiac filling (18). Ruffmann et al. (19) found that a higher left ventricular mass/volume ratio and a lower peak velocity of early diastolic filling are associated with a higher incidence of intradialytic hypotension. A decrease in venous compliance, as observed in hypertensive dialysis patients, leads to an even steeper fall in ventricular filling pressure when circulating blood volume decreases (20).

Combined ultrafiltration-hemodialysis is known to result in a decrease in venous tone measured at the forearm, which further impairs cardiac filling (21,22). In agreement, Chaignon et al. (23) showed that combined ultrafiltration-hemodialysis results in a decentralization of blood volume. In contrast, and probably on the basis of a lower extracorporeal blood temperature, both isolated ultrafiltration and hemofiltration are associated with a clear increase in venous tone, thus maintaining cardiac filling pressures more adequately (24). Therefore, either sequential ultrafiltration-hemodialysis or hemofiltration could be used in patients who frequently suffer from hemodynamic instability on the basis of severe diastolic dysfunction. Another option in these patients might be to change from intermittent dialysis to CAPD, which is associated with smaller and more gradual changes in intravascular volume.

Therapeutic Options

Therapeutic measures in relation to the dialysis treatment itself should aim at a reduction of chronic pressure and volume overload while reducing plasma levels of uremic toxins related to LVH. In this respect, CAPD patients might benefit from the absence of an arteriovenous fistula (9) and a somewhat higher clearance of middle molecules. However, although there are no controlled studies in which patient selection is excluded, the incidence of cardiovascular mortality and morbidity between patients treated with hemodialysis and those undergoing CAPD is in general the same, suggesting no specific advantage of either therapy (1). Hüting et al. (25) found an incidence of LVH of 84% in a cohort of 55 normotensive CAPD patients. In addition, both a decrease (26) and an increase in LV mass have been observed in patients while on CAPD. In addition, again in CAPD patients, LVH has been related to control of arterial blood pressure (27).

Improving clearance of uremic toxins in general could lead to a reduction of the need for rhEPO in treating anemia. Correction of anemia by rhEPO treatment has been shown to result in a reduction of left ventricular mass indices and diameter (28–30). Moreover, different authors also found a reduction of the hyperdynamic state characterized by a decrease in global systolic function and heart rate and an increase in peripheral resistance (28,31). In the long term, arterial blood pressure seems to be unaffected by the increase in hematocrit (32). With respect to clearance, renal replacement therapies such as hemofiltration and hemodiafiltration could be of benefit in patients with LVH. To our knowledge no studies have been published regarding this specific possibility. Although the relationship has not been studied recently, the pioneers of convective dialysis treatments have claimed better control of severe hypertension with hemofiltration, which could influence LVH (33). Quellhorst et al. (34) found a lower hospitalization rate in relation to hypotension, hypertension, and myocardial disease and a higher survival rate in a group of patients more than 60 years old treated with hemofiltration as compared to those treated with hemodialysis or CAPD. Also, in relation to the suggested role of hyperparathyroidism in the development of uremic cardiomyopathy (2), a higher clearance of PTH might result in a reduction of LVH.

Control of blood pressure seems to be an important goal in reducing LVH. Pascual et al. (29) found that left ventricular mass remained significantly higher in a group of hypertensive dialysis patients after correction of anemia as compared to a group of normotensive patients not using antihypertensive medication. Moreover, Canella et al. (35) showed that long-term (24 months) treatment of

hypertension with ACE inhibitors, beta-blockers and calcium antagonists resulted in a decline of the interventricular septum thickness
and left ventricular mass to a degree observed in spontaneous normotensive uremic patients. To get more insight into the relationship
between the dialysis treatment itself and both hypertension and cardiac structure, we recently compared 22 patients from our center
treated with bicarbonate hemodialysis three times a week for 3–4
hours (Kt/V 1.1 ± 0.2) with 26 patients from the dialysis center in
Tassin treated with acetate hemodialysis three times a week for 8
hours (Kt/V 1.8 ± 0.4). The patients from Tassin are known to have
a low incidence of hypertension and a better survival that might be
related to a higher clearance of small and middle molecules or to
their relative hypovolemic state (36). Seventy-three percent of our
patients were using antihypertensive medication, and both arterial
blood pressure [(143 ± 26)/(81 ± 16)] and pulse pressure (ambulatory, 48 hours) were significantly higher than in the patients from
Tassin [(115 ± 21)/(67 ± 11)], none of whom used antihypertensive
medication. This difference could not be explained on the basis of
differences in volume status as measured by the inferior caval vein
diameter. However, both groups had a comparable degree of sym-
metrical LVH, while systolic and diastolic function were equally disturbed as compared to a group of normotensive, age-matched controls without renal disease.

The difference in arterial blood pressure between our patients
and those from Tassin was explained on the basis of a significantly
higher level of calculated systemic vascular resistance in our patients
despite the use of antihypertensive medication such as ACE inhibitors and calcium antagonists. Of all measured parameters, only hematocrit was significantly higher in our patients (34 ± 6 vs. 30 ± 5%),
and only in the Tassin patients was the LVM index inversely correlated with hematocrit ($r = -0.44; p < 0.05$) (37).

In both healthy controls and the Tassin patients, we also evaluated arterial compliance and distensibility by Doppler analysis of the
vessel wall movements. As compared to the control group, femoral
artery distensibility and compliance were lower in the patients on
long-treatment-time dialysis, although only the latter reached statistical significance. There were, however, no differences in carotid

artery distensibility or compliance (unpublished data). At variance, Barenbrock et al. (38) found a decrease in the distensibility of the common carotid artery, studying 24 normotensive (<140/90) dialysis patients not using antihypertensive medication who were treated with hemodialysis three times a week for 3–5 hours. London et al. (39), in a study of ESRD patients, found an increase in aortic pulse wave velocity indicative of an increase in aortic stiffness that could not be explained on the basis of age, blood pressure, retention of uremic waste products, or lipid abnormalities.

Thus, despite a very low incidence of hypertension in patients on long-treatment-time dialysis, they still suffer from LVH and cardiac dysfunction as observed in hypertensive dialysis patients. This contrasts with the results obtained by Canella et al. (35), who found a definite regression of LVH with aggressive antihypertensive treatment. However, patients from Tassin had a lower hematocrit than our patients, while the femoral artery elastic properties were impaired as compared to healthy controls, which further stresses the importance of these two factors in the development of LVH.

CONCLUSIONS

With the results obtained from the present studies, it is still very difficult to define the factors responsible for normotension in long-treatment-time dialysis with a high Kt/V. It is also unknown whether a higher clearance of middle molecules could be of importance in relation to the treatment of hypertension, the regression of LVH, and long-term outcome. Finally, the relationship between different aspects of the uremic state and arterial compliance should be further determined. Therefore, prospective studies controlled for anemia are necessary to further define the importance of these factors and their possible interaction in relation to the cardiovascular system.

REFERENCES

1. Raine AEG, Margreiter R, Brunner FP, Ehrich JHH, Geerlings W, Landais P, Loiret C, Mallick NP, Selwood NH, Tufveson, Valderrabano F.

Report on management of renal failure in Europe, XXII, 1991. Nephrol Dialysis Transplant 1992; 7:7–35.

2. Harnett JD, Parfrey PS, Griffiths SM, Gault MH, Barre P, Guttmann RD. Left ventricular hypertrophy in end-stage renal disease. Nephron 1988; 48:107–115.

3. Foley RN, Parfrey PS, Harnett JD, Kent GM, Martin CJ, Murray DC, Barre PE. Clinical and echographic disease in patients starting with end-stage renal disease therapy. Kidney Int 1995; 47:186–192.

4. Parfrey PS, Harnett JD, Griffiths SM, Taylor R, Hand J, King A, Barre PE. The clinical course of left ventricular hypertrophy in dialysis patients. Nephron 1990; 55:114–120.

5. Hüting J, Kramer W, Schütterle, Wizemann V. Analysis of left-ventriclar changes associated with chronic hemodialysis. Nephron 1988; 49: 284–290.

6. Silberberg JS, Barre PE, Prichard SS, Sniderman AD. Impact of left ventricular hypertrophy on survival in end-stage renal disease. Kidney Int 1989; 36:286–290.

7. Casale PN, Devereux RB, Milner M, Zullo G, Harshfield GA, Pickering TG, Laragh JH. Value of echocardiographic measurements of left ventricular mass in predicting cardiovascular morbid events in hypertensive men. Ann Intern Med 1986; 105:173–187.

8. Foley RN, Parfrey PS, Harnett JD. Left ventricular hypertrophy in dialysis patients. Sem Dialysis 1992; 5:34–41.

9. London GM, Marchais SJ, Guerin AP, Metivier F, Pannier B. Cardiac hypertrophy and arterial alterations in end-stage renal disease: hemodynamic factors. Kidney Int 1993; 43:S42–S49.

10. Rambausek M, Ritz E, Mall G, Mehls O, Katus H. Myocardial hypertrophy in rats with renal insufficiency. Kidney Int 1985; 28:775–778.

11. Mall G, Rambausek M, Neumeister A, Kollmar S, Vetterlein F, Ritz E. Myocardial interstitial fibrosis in experimental uremia—implications for cardiac compliance. Kidney Int 1988; 33:804–811.

12. Ritz E, Rambausek M, Mall G, Ruffmann K, Mandelbaum A. Cardiac changes in uremia and their possible relation to cardiovascular instability on dialysis. Contrib Nephrol 1990; 78:221–229.

13. Mall G, Huther W, Schneider J, Lundin P, Ritz E. Diffuse intramyocardiocytic fibrosis in uraemic patients. Nephrol Dialysis Transplant 1990; 5:39–44.

14. London GM, Fabiani F, Marchais SJ, De Vernejoul M-C, Guerin AP, Safar ME, Metivier F, Llach F. Uremic cardiomyopathy: an inadequate ventricular hypertrophy. Kidney Int 1987; 31:973–980.

15. Symons C, Fortune F, Greenbaum RA, Dandone P. Cardiac hypertro- phy, hypertrophic cardiomyopathy and hyperparathyroidism: an asso- ciation. Br Heart J 1985; 54:539–542.
16. Greaves SC, Gamble GD, Collins JF, Whalley GA, Sharpe DN. Deter- minants of left ventricular hypertrophy and systolic dysfunction in chronic renal failure. Am J Kidney Dis 1994; 24:768–776.
17. Harnett JD, Kent GM, Barre PE, Taylor R, Parfrey PS. Risk factors for the development of left ventricular hypertrophy in a prospectively followed cohort of dialysis patients. J Am Soc Nephrol 1994; 4:1486– 1490.
18. Kramer W, Wizemann V, Lammlein G, Thormann J, Kindler M, Schelpper M, Schütterle G. Cardiac dysfunction in patients on main- tenance hemodialysis. II: Systolic and diastolic properties of the left ventricle assessed by invasive methods. Contrib Nephrol 1986; 52:110– 124.
19. Ruffmann K, Mandelbaum A, Bommer J, Schmidli M, Ritz E. Doppler echocardiographic findings in dialysis patients. Nephrol Dialysis Trans- plant 1990; 5:426–431.
20. Kooman JP, Wijnen JAG, Draaijer P, van Bortel LMAB, Gladziwa U, Peltenburg HG, Struyker-Boudier HAJ, van Hooff JP, Leunissen KML. Compliance and reactivity of the peripheral venous system in chronic intermittent hemodialysis. Kidney Int 1992; 41:1041–1048.
21. Bradley JR, Evans DB, Cowley AJ. Comparison of vascular tone during combined haemodialysis with ultrafiltration and during ultrafiltration followed by haemodialysis: a possible mechanism for dialysis hypoten- sion. Br Med J 1990; 300:1312.
22. Kooman JP, Gladziwa U, Böcker G, van Bortel LMAB, van Hooff JP, Leunissen KML. Role of the venous system in hemodynamics during ultrafiltration and bicarbonate dialysis. Kidney Int 1992; 42:718–726.
23. Chaignon M, Tzuoh Chen W, Tarazi RC, Bravo EL, Nakamoto S. Ef- fect of hemodialysis on blood volume distribution and cardiac output. Hypertension 1981; 3:327–332.
24. van Kuijk WHM, Luik AJ, de Leeuw PW, van Hooff JP, Nieman FHM, Habets HML, Leunissen KML. Vascular reactivity during hemodia- lysis and isolated ultrafiltration: thermal influences. Nephrol Dialysis Transplant 1995; 10:1852–1858.
25. Hüting J, Kramer W, Reitinger J, Kuhn K, Wizemann V, Schtterle G. Cardiac structure and function in continuous ambulatory peritoneal dialysis: influence of blood purification and hypercirculation. Am Heart J 1990; 119:344–352.

26. Leenen FH, Smith DL, Khanna R, Oreopoulos DG. Changes in left ventricular hypertrophy and function in hypertensive patients started on continuous ambulatory peritoneal dialaysis. Am Heart J 1985; 110: 102–106.

27. Huting J, Alpert MA. Progression of left ventricular hypertrophy in end-stage renal disease treated by continuous ambulatory peritoneal dialysis depends on hypertension and hypercirculation. Clin Cardiol 1992; 15:190–196.

28. London GM, Zins B, Pannier B, Naret C, Berthelot J-M, Jacquot C, Safar M, Drueke TB. Vascular changes in hemodialysis patients in response to recombinant human erythropoietin. Kidney Int 1989; 36: 878–882.

29. Pascual J, Teruel JL, Moya JL, Liaño F, Jiménez-Mena M, Ortuño J. Regression of left ventricular hypertrophy after partial correction of anemia with erythropoietin in patients on hemodialysis: a prospective study. Clin Nephrol 1991; 35:280–287.

30. Canella G, La Canna G, Sandrini M, Gaggiotti M, Nordio G, Movilli E, Mombelloni S, Visioli O, Maiorca R. Reversal of left ventricular hypertrophy following recombinant human erythropoietin treatment of anaemic dialysed uraemic patients. Nephrol Dialysis Transplant 1991; 6:31–37.

31. Fellner SK, Lang RM, Neumann A, Korcarz C, Borow KM. Cardiovascular consequences of correction of the anemia of renal failure with erythropoietin. Kidney Int 1993; 44:1309–1315.

32. Wirtz JJJM, Leunissen KML, van Kiujk W, Cheriex EC, Slaaf DW, Reneman RS, van Hooff JP. Long-term effects of recombinant human erythropoietin on macro- and microcirculation in chronic hemnodialysis patients. Blood Purif 1993; 11:237–247.

33. Quellhorst E, Doht B, Schuenemann B. Hemofiltration: treatment of renal failure by ultrafiltration and substitution. J Dialysis 1977; 1:529–543.

34. Quellhorst EA, Schuenemann B, Mietzsch G. Long-term hemofiltration in "poor risk" patients. Trans Am Soc Artif Intern Organs 1987; 33:758–764.

35. Canella G, Paoletti E, Delfino R, Peloso G, Molinari S, Traverso GB. Regression of left ventricular hypertrophy in hypertensive uremic patients on long-term antihypertensive therapy. Kidney Int 1993; 44:881–886.

36. Charra B, Calemard E, Ruffet M, Chazot C, Terrat JC, Vanel T, Laurent G. Survival as an index of adequacy of dialysis. Kidney Int 1992; 41:1286–1291.

37. Luik AJ, Charra B, Katzarski K, Habets J, Cheriex EC, Laurent G, Bergström J, Leunissen KML. Blood pressure control and fluid state in patients on long treatment time dialysis [abstr]. J Am Soc Nephrol 1994; 5:521.
38. Barenbrock M, Spieker C, Laske V, Heidenreich S, Hohage H, Bachmann J, Hoeks APG, Rahn K-H. Studies of the vessel wall properties in hemodialysis patients. Kidney Int 1994; 45:1397–1400.
39. London G, Marchais SJ, Safar ME, Genest AF, Guerin AP, Metivier F, Chedid K, London AM. Aortic and large artery compliance in end-stage renal failure. Kidney Int 1990; 37:137–142.

11

Evidence-Based Recommendations for the Clinical Use of rhEPO

N. Muirhead   University of Western Ontario, London, Ontario, Canada

INTRODUCTION

The introduction of recombinant human erythropoietin (rhEPO) into clinical practice has fundamentally altered the way in which the anemia of chronic renal failure is managed. Utilization of rhEPO worldwide (1–3) has reached a point at which, in some countries at least, the majority of dialysis patients are receiving this therapy (Table 1). However, with some 10 years having elapsed since the initial reports of clinical use of rhEPO for renal anemia, it is time to examine critically the evidence on which such widespread use of rhEPO is based. That is the purpose of this chapter.

THE MORBIDITY OF RENAL ANEMIA

Anemia is an almost inevitable consequence of chronic renal failure, and, while many factors have been implicated in its pathogenesis

Table 1   rhEPO Utilization by Country (1993)

	Hemodialysis (%)	Peritoneal dialysis (%)
Austria	77	60
Belgium	83	71
Denmark	72	55
France	45	56
Germany (West)	57	49
Italy	47	33
Norway	83	40
Poland	51	49
Spain	57	39
Sweden	85	54
Switzerland	74	55
United Kingdom	53	34
Canada	59	47
United States[a]	88	52

[a]U.S. figures are for 1992.
Source: Refs. 1–3.

(Table 2), it is now abundantly clear that deficiency of erythropoietin (EPO) is by far the most important cause (4). Many symptoms experienced by uremic patients, such as fatigue, poor exercise tolerance, and dyspnea, are related to anemia. Some conditions such as angina or peripheral vascular disease may be aggravated by anemia. It is also clear from observations made in patients receiving rhEPO that many of the symptoms previously ascribed to uremia, including sleep disturbance, sexual dysfunction, and cognitive impairment, are also, at least in part, related to anemia (5–11).

The morbidity associated with such complaints is substantial, but would not be expected to have a major impact on mortality. However, anemia has recently been identified as a leading risk factor for the development of left ventricular hypertrophy (LVH) in patients with end-stage renal disease (ESRD) (12). LVH, in turn, has been identified as a leading predictor of cardiac morbidity and mortality among ESRD patients that is independent of age, diabetes, congestive heart failure, ischemic heart disease, hypertension, or hypoalbuminemia (12). The expectation that relief of anemia with rhEPO

Table 2 Causes of Anemia
in Renal Failure

Erythropoietin deficiency
Hemolysis
Iron deficiency
Deficiency of other hematinics
Gastrointestinal blood loss
Dialysis-related blood loss
Iatrogenic
Aluminum overload

might prevent the development of, or allow regression of, LVH (13) has been one of the major driving forces for the widespread use of rhEPO. An examination of the appropriateness of this strategy will be presented below, based on evidence available in the literature.

In many countries, decisions regarding the use of rhEPO seem to have been made in response to political or economic pressures, rather than clinical need or expectation of benefit. This is the readiest explanation for the wide discrepancies between countries in rhEPO utilization (Table 1). One of the objectives of this chapter is to provide a rational basis for clinical decision-making regarding rhEPO use. Such an approach may be useful in persuading third-party payers, i.e., government in most jurisdictions, to provide financial support for rhEPO therapy.

CLINICAL BENEFITS OF rhEPO

Existing therapies for renal anemia prior to the advent of rhEPO therapy were limited both in their ability to produce stable anemia correction and by their tendency to cause significant side effects. Androgen therapy is associated with virilization and risk of liver disease (14,15), while blood transfusion carries risks of viral infections, allosensitization, and iron overload (16,17). An alternative to these treatments that would permit stable anemia correction with minimal side effects is seen as highly desirable by most nephrologists.

Clinical trials in a variety of ESRD populations—hemodialysis, continuous ambulatory peritoneal dialysis (CAPD), predialysis, and failing renal allograft—indicate that rhEPO produces a predictable, dose-dependent increase in hemoglobin, although the extent of any associated clinical benefit is difficult to determine, given the heterogeneity of study designs and outcomes. This had led to problems in generalizing results of clinical trials to individual clinical practice, and has prompted at least one distinguished investigator in the field to express concern regarding the failure of rhEPO to live up to its initial promise (18).

Benefits that have been ascribed to rhEPO therapy in clinical trials include improvement in quality of life (QOL), exercise capacity, sexual function, and cognitive ability, and reduced hospitalization. These benefits have been noted, to some extent, in all ESRD populations studied to date. However, the acceptance of such trial data requires a critical examination of the quality of the evidence provided, so that an objective decision regarding the place of rhEPO in clinical practice can be reached.

THE EVIDENCE-BASED APPROACH

The development of rhEPO is, by itself, an interesting example of the complexities of introducing new and expensive biotechnology products into clinical medicine (19). It is undeniable that rhEPO is expensive, and likely to remain so. The world market for rhEPO, at least in the ESRD area, will remain very small relative to huge markets such as those for hypertension and diabetes therapies. Given the high development and production costs for an agent that has a limited market, it is not surprising that it should remain expensive. This problem is not confined to rhEPO but is seen with other biotechnology products such as G-CSF and even t-PA, despite its vastly larger potential market.

These economic facts of life, coupled with very real concerns by governments worldwide about escalating health-care costs, are driving physicians to be much more cost-conscious and critical when evaluating new or established therapies. These concerns are at the heart of the current drive toward evidence-based medicine (20,21), quite apart from any desire to identify the best therapies for our patients. A number of potential approaches can be used to assess the quality of evidence regarding new therapies. The approach taken in this chapter is modeled after the levels of evidence defined by Carruthers et al. (22). Papers were classified according to criteria defined for papers regarding therapy, quality assurance, and prevention using the following scheme:

1. Randomized control trial (RCT) of adequate sample size.
2. An RCT not meeting level 1 criteria
3. Non-RCT with contemporaneous controls selected by a systematic process; subgroup analysis of an RCT
4. Before/after study or case series of >10 patients with historical controls.
5. Case series of >10 patients
6. Case series of <10 patients

Review articles were also included and classified as level 1 (evidence of a comprehensive search for evidence, avoidance of bias in selecting studies, assessment of validity for each study cited, and conclusions supported by the data and analysis presented) or level 2 (presence of any three of the above criteria). The quality of the published evidence was evaluated for predialysis, hemodialysis, peritoneal dialysis, and failing allograft patients.

rhEPO IN PREDIALYSIS PATIENTS

There have been relatively few large-scale studies of rhEPO in predialysis patients. Of those that have been published, only two meet level 1 or 2 criteria, as defined, and the remainder are small studies with heterogeneous study designs and/or outcomes that meet level 4 criteria or less. The U.S. multicenter study (23) is a level 1 placebo-controlled trial of various intravenous (i.v.) rhEPO doses in 117 predialysis patients. This study found evidence for a dose-response relationship similar to that encountered in hemodialysis patients, and significant improvements in energy levels and work capacity in patients who had their anemia corrected. No significant increase in the occurrence or severity of high blood pressure was noted for rhEPO patients compared to those taking placebo. There was no evidence over the short (3 months) placebo comparison period of any more rapid deterioration in renal function in patients receiving rhEPO. The Austrian multicenter study (24) examined the response to subcutaneous (s.c.) rhEPO in 123 patients, with no placebo comparison, over a 3-month period. Again, a satisfactory hemoglobin increase was achieved in the majority of patients, with few adverse effects and no impact on the rate of decline in renal function.

The remaining studies are either too small or too limited in experimental design (e.g., lack of placebo controls) to add any meaningful data. However, the benefits proposed for hemodialysis patients, such as improvement in QOL, exercise capacity, and cognitive function, are hinted at in these studies (25–28). One cautionary note for the predialysis patient is the lingering uncertainty concerning the effect of rhEPO therapy on progression of renal failure. Published studies, including the U.S. multicenter study, do not indicate a more rapid rate of decline in renal function during rhEPO therapy, despite concerns raised in animal studies. However, it must be noted that the duration of rhEPO therapy in most of these studies, including the placebo-controlled U.S. study, was only 3 months. Failure to identify an effect of rhEPO therapy on progression of renal failure may well be the result of the relatively brief period of observation in published studies. At least one recent study (29), as yet unpublished, suggests that longer periods of rhEPO therapy in predialysis patients may lead to a more rapid rate of decline in renal function. This is an area that will require further study in a larger trial with an appropriate observation period.

rhEPO IN HEMODIALYSIS PATIENTS

Surprisingly, of all the studies published on the use of rhEPO in hemodialysis patients, only one—the Canadian multicenter study (9)—meets level 1 criteria. Both the U.S. (8) and the European (7) multicenter studies meet only level 3 criteria because of their lack of a placebo comparison group, despite their large size. Studies in hemo-dialysis patients were the first to be published on the use of rhEPO for renal anemia and, as such, the first to demonstrate the dose-re-sponse relationship and to establish the expected levels of anemia correction (5,6). The Canadian study examined QOL and exercise capacity, and found that both improved after rhEPO therapy com-pared to placebo, in parallel with the degree of anemia correction (9). Long-term follow-up was unable to detect clinically important differences in these outcomes for patients with higher hemoglobins (30). The European multicenter study confirmed the efficacy and relative safety of rhEPO therapy (7). The U.S. cooperative study demonstrated reductions in overall morbidity and hospitalizations, as well as confirming efficacy (8).

All these studies added to data concerning adverse effects of rhEPO therapy and have had a major impact on prescribing habits for rhEPO. An overall 33% rate of de novo development of hyper-tension, or aggravation of existing hypertension, was reported in these studies. Early concerns regarding seizure (31,32) were largely dis-counted by the placebo-controlled study. Other adverse events have been uncommon or minor, except for a tendency toward an increased rate of access clotting and replacement (33,34), specifically for syn-thetic arteriovenous grafts (30,35,36).

The body of evidence for rhEPO in hemodialysis patients sug-gests strongly that anemia can be improved in over 90% of patients with an acceptably low incidence of serious side effects. Benefits that have been shown to accrue from this treatment include improved QOL, physical endurance, and exercise capacity. Hospital days and readmission rates are lower for patients with hematocrits over 30% (3,37), while some studies have suggested that rhEPO use may be associated with cost savings (38–40).

rhEPO IN PERITONEAL DIALYSIS PATIENTS

In contrast to the situation with studies in hemodialysis patients, there are comparatively few published studies of rhEPO in peritoneal di-alysis patients. There have been no level 1 RCTs and only one RCT meeting level 2 criteria (41). The majority of studies have been small or of limited duration and thus meet only level 4 or 5 criteria. The single relevant RCT examined issues of efficacy and safety rather than QOL, exercise capacity, or other clinical outcomes, which have been examined only in the smaller studies indicated above. The U.S. multicenter study found efficacy and adverse-event profiles to be similar to those encountered in hemodialysis patients (41). However, the relatively short duration of the placebo comparison period (12 weeks) does not permit a more detailed comparison of QOL or other clinical benefits. Several small studies have reported improvement in QOL and cognitive function in CAPD patients (42,43) as well as improvements in exercise and nutritional status (44,45).

Minor changes in peritoneal membrane-transport characteristics have been reported during rhEPO therapy. The most consistent observation has been a switch to "low transporter" type. The effect is small and of, as yet, unknown clinical significance. This is clearly an area for further study in peritoneal dialysis patients.

rhEPO IN RENAL TRANSPLANT PATIENTS

Anemia is common in patients experiencing chronic renal allograft failure and probably contributes significantly to morbidity. Several small studies have examined the use of rhEPO in such patients (46, 47). All are level 4 or 5 studies. The consistent finding has been that— despite concomitant immunosuppressive therapy, including the use of azathioprine—the efficacy and dose requirements are similar to those encountered in other ESRD populations. Clinical benefits such as improved QOL have also proved to be similar. One study (47) suggested that the rate of decline in renal function accelerated during rhEPO therapy. Other studies have not found this to be the case. However, all the studies are either too small or of too short a duration to provide a definitive answer to this concern. This is clearly an additional area for further study.

The ability of rhEPO therapy to enhance renal transplant outcome by reducing the degree of allosensitization has also been studied. Again, the studies reported are small and of short duration.

However, several authors have reported a significant reduction in the degree of allosensitization in previously transfused patients during rhEPO therapy (48,49). Several studies have examined the impact of hematocrit at the time of transplant on renal allograft function. The studies are small and the results hard to interpret. One study suggested an increased rate of delayed graft function at hematocrits >30% (50) while two small studies (51,52) found no such association. Given the widespread use of rhEPO in dialysis patients and the increased interest in higher hematocrits (53), based on the potential for cardiac benefit (vide infra), the issue of whether a higher hemoglobin at the time of transplant has a deleterious effect on renal allograft function requires further clarification.

GUIDELINES FOR THE CLINICAL USE OF rhEPO

In developing guidelines for the optimal use of rhEPO, a number of key questions must be answered:

1. Who should receive rhEPO?
2. How should patients be selected?
3. What is the best route of rhEPO administration?
4. What is the correct dose of rhEPO?
5. What are the pros and cons of rhEPO therapy?
6. What should the target hemoglobin be?

For some of these questions, clear data are available in the literature that guide the choices that clinicians make. For others, a considerable amount of intuition or "clinical judgment" must be used.

Who Should Receive rhEPO?

The data in the literature indicate that almost all patients with anemia caused by renal failure can expect an increase in hemoglobin of at least 20 g/L in response to rhEPO therapy (7–9,23,24,41,47). The simplest answer to this question is thus that all patients with anemia related to renal failure should receive rhEPO. However, this response ignores the adverse events associated with rhEPO use, particularly the risk of dialysis access failure, as well as the expected clinical benefits. In most parts of the world, the decisions on who will receive rhEPO seem to be made largely on the basis of fiscal rather than clinical considerations. In the United States, where Medicare picks up the cost of rhEPO (54) provided that an arbitrary hematocrit cutoff (currently 36%) is not exceeded, almost all dialysis patients are on rhEPO. In Canada, on the other hand, there is wide variability in the willingness of provincial health budgets to pay for rhEPO, thus producing wide discrepancies (3) in rhEPO utilization across the country (Table 3).

With so much of the clinical decision-making being influenced by fiscal concerns, the situation for predialysis and failing allograft patients is even less uncertain. Given that the data concerning the use of rhEPO in such patients are less strong than for dialysis patients, at present it is not possible to recommend that rhEPO be used routinely for such patients.

How Should Patients Be Selected?

Ideally, patients should be selected for rhEPO therapy based on their ability to achieve meaningful clinical benefits in areas such as QOL and exercise capacity, rather than on the presence of anemia alone.

Table 3   Regional Variation in rhEPO Utilization in Canada

	Hemodialysis (%)	Peritoneal dialysis (%)
Canada	58.8	46.7
Newfoundland	42.4	42.6
Nova Scotia/P.E.I.	26.1	37.2
New Brunswick	61.1	42.9
Quebec	56.4	36.9
Ontario	69.9	56.8
Manitoba	30.0	39.7
Saskatchewan	50.0	32.1
Alberta	49.2	43.1
British Columbia	66.8	39.0

Source: Data from 1993 Canadian Organ Replacement Registry (3).

However, it should be obvious from the wide variability in rhEPO utilization data that unless physicians in different countries differ widely in their understanding of the clinical benefits of rhEPO, decisions are rarely made on this basis. This, indeed, may be at the heart of Dr. Eschbach's recent frustration (18).

In terms of hard evidence, rhEPO therapy should be limited to patients who can expect to derive clinical benefit. This will include patients capable of achieving a meaningful improvement in QOL, those in whom anemia-related symptoms are expected to decline, and those for whom avoidance of blood transfusion is desirable. Careful selection of patients likely to benefit (Table 4) would be expected to maximize the cost-effectiveness of rhEPO therapy.

What Is the Best Route of rhEPO Administration?

The early studies of rhEPO were conducted in hemodialysis patients, and the i.v. route of administration was both convenient and effective (5–9). Later studies have indicated that s.c. rhEPO administration is

Table 4   Evidence-Based Criteria for rhEPO Therapy

1. Anemia related to erythropoietin deficiency
   a. Implies exclusion of other causes
   b. Implies correction of iron deficiency in advance
2. Presence of symptoms felt to be due to anemia, e.g., fatigue, diminished exercise tolerance
3. Underlying disease state aggravated by anemia
   a. Active cardiac ischemia
   b. Congestive heart failure
4. Reasonable expectation of *clinical* benefit, e.g., patient *not* bedridden or confined to a wheelchair
5. Avoidance of transfusions/androgens clinically desirable
   a. Risk of allosensitization (e.g., *awaiting* transplant)
   b. Fear of viral transmission
   c. Current iron overload
   d. Severe transfusion reactions
   e. Contraindication to androgens
6. For predialysis patients
   a. Evidence of stable renal function in the 3 months prior to rhEPO therapy
   b. Risk of decline in renal function related to baseline function

as effective as i.v., but that dose requirements are, on the average, 30–50% less (55–57). Concerns that s.c. rhEPO would be too painful are probably unfounded. In one study in which s.c. and i.v. administration were compared, complaints of pain following s.c. administration were actually more common during administration of placebo (55). The s.c. route is the only practical route for outpatient rhEPO administration, e.g., in CAPD or predialysis patients. Intraperitoneal administration of rhEPO in CAPD patients requires larger doses unless it can be given into the dry peritoneal cavity (58). It is thus recommended that rhEPO be given by s.c. administration to all patients unless there are compelling reasons (e.g., coagulopathy) to avoid the s.c. route.

What Is the Correct Dose of rhEPO?

The earliest studies of rhEPO indicated that there was a clear dose-response relationship. Doses of up to 500 mg/kg body weight three times weekly were used in these studies (5,6). Subsequent studies have used much lower starting doses (usually 50–100 μg/kg three times weekly), which are equally effective at producing a satisfactory hemoglobin response and have a much lower incidence of serious side effects, particularly hypertension and seizures (7–9). The current recommendation, based on the expectation that over 90% of patients will have an increase in hemoglobin by >20 g/L during the first 12 weeks of treatment, is that rhEPO be begun at a dose of 50 μg/kg three times weekly s.c.

Dose frequency is a rather more contentious issue, and has been studied poorly. The evidence available do suggest, however, that with i.v. rhEPO the dose frequency usually cannot be decreased (59). In contrast, a significant fraction of patients receiving s.c. rhEPO can have their dose frequency decreased (60,61). The majority of patients require s.c. rhEPO once or twice weekly, while occasional patients require much less frequent rhEPO administration.

What Are the Pros and Cons of rhEPO Therapy?

Much of the data in the literature focus, not surprisingly, on the benefits of rhEPO therapy. However, for any new therapy to be worthwhile, it should preferably be safer, more effective, and less expensive than prior therapies. In this context, rhEPO might not, at first glance, fare very well. Despite the clinical benefits of rhEPO therapy, there are significant adverse effects, especially hypertension (7–9,62) and access failure (30,33–35). The drug remains expensive, even if the s.c. route of administration is used. The patients for whom evidence of the cost-effectiveness of rhEPO therapy is available (38) represent only a small fraction of those on dialysis. It is not possible to generalize the results of studies in such patients to the ESRD population as a whole, although utilization data suggest that this is exactly what has happened in some countries.

However, there is no doubt that, for carefully selected patients, rhEPO therapy is safe, clinically beneficial, and cost-effective (38, 39,63). The adverse effects of rhEPO therapy are predictable and can be avoided by the prudent clinician. Avoidance of too rapid an increase in hemoglobin and careful attention to blood-pressure control can eliminate concerns about hypertension and seizures (9,64). Vigilance with regard to early warnings of impending access problems, e.g., rising venous pressures (65), plus judicious use of antiplatelet drugs and anticoagulants can diminish the threat of access failure (66). Despite concerns to the contrary (67), there are no convincing data that rhEPO therapy impairs hemodialysis efficiency (8, 9,55), or that it accelerates the rate of decline in renal function in predialysis patients (23,24).

What Should the Target Hemoglobin Be?

This issue remains unresolved. The majority of clinical trials on which current clinical practices are based used hemoglobin targets in the range of 100–130 g/L. All the data concerning QOL, exercise capacity, and other clinical benefits of rhEPO have thus been derived from studies with hemoglobin targets that represent less than full correction of anemia (7–9). Advocates of higher hemoglobin targets suggest that higher targets will inevitably mean more clinical benefit. A particular point has been made of the relationship between correction of anemia and regression of LVH, and the potential for this to have a beneficial impact on cardiovascular morbidity and mortality.

Certainly, data from a number of studies (13,68–76) suggest that there is a benefit to be gained from even partial anemia correction in allowing regression of LVH (Table 5). However, this does not necessarily mean that more complete or prolonged correction will allow further benefits to accrue. In this context, it should be pointed out that although the only placebo-controlled RCT in hemodialysis patients found that QOL improved further as hemoglobin rose, adverse events were also more frequent at the higher hemoglobin levels (9).

Economics is another factor that, unfortunately, must be considered. Powe et al. (54) have estimated, using Medicare data, that the incremental costs of rhEPO would add some 6% ($590 million U.S.) to the annual Medicare budget after 5 years. This assumes Medicare reimbursement for rhEPO to a hematocrit target of 33%. This target has already been revised upward to 36%. The incremental costs of moving to an even higher hematocrit target, closer to normal (e.g., 40%), are currently unknown as there are no data concerning the dose of rhEPO required to provide this level of anemia correction. However, it seems likely that the required dose, and hence costs, will be even higher than those mentioned above.

Table 5   Effect of rhEPO on Left Ventricular Mass

Investigator	n	Mean Δ Hb (g/L)	Mean Δ LV mass (%)
Zehnder et al. (68)	12	19	−34.5
Low-Friedrich et al. (69)	25	24	−11.0
Canella et al. (70)	9	43	−32.2
Silberberg (13)	22	51	−15.0
Goldberg et al. (71)	15	33	−39.8
Macdougall et al. (72)	10	44	−26.1
Martinez-Vea et al. (73)	9	35	−25.2
London et al. (74)	11	38	−17.4
Pascual et al. (75)	15	41	−34.0
Wizemann et al. (76)	28	41	−19.6
Totals	156	37.9	−25.5

In terms only of clinical outcomes for which objective clinical trial data are available, there is no justification for recommending a target hemoglobin in excess of 110 g/L at present. The issue is further complicated by the question of who receives rhEPO. In Canada, the average drug-acquisition costs for patients receiving s.c. rhEPO are around $500 Canadian annually. There is evidence that a cost of this order represents the break-even point for cost-effectiveness of rhEPO for hemodialysis patients (38). For predialysis patients, the potential to defer dialysis through an improvement in well-being following rhEPO use may more than offset the costs of therapy. However, there are no objective data that such an outcome is possible. To date, the issue of cost-effectiveness of rhEPO has been addressed only to a limited extent for hemodialysis patients (38,39,63,77), and not at all for other ESRD populations. Additional data will be required before a firm target hemoglobin level can be set because the target will need to be a pragmatic blend of the clinically desirable and economically feasible.

FINAL RECOMMENDATIONS

At present, there is evidence that partial correction of anemia with rhEPO is accompanied by measurable clinical benefits, notably in the areas of QOL and exercise tolerance. For hemodialysis patients, the data are convincing. rhEPO should thus be offered to all hemodialysis patients for whom there is a reasonable expectation that the clinical benefits noted above can occur. For CAPD patients, the clinical trials have not been large enough or long enough in duration to generate meaningful data. However, the data that are available show benefits similar to those seen in hemodialysis patients. It is thus recommended that use of rhEPO in CAPD patients proceed in a fashion similar to that in hemodialysis patients. As further clinical trial data become available from CAPD patients, this view may need to be modified. Data for predialysis patients suggest that the use of rhEPO is safe, and could be cost-effective if it leads to a delay in dialysis start because of the elimination of anemia-related symptoms. However, the lack of any lengthy placebo-comparison study, and the mixed results of studies examining the effect of rhEPO on the rate of decline in renal failure, suggest that caution should be exercised regarding the use of rhEPO in both predialysis and failing allograft patients. Routine use of rhEPO for anemia is thus not recommended in either group.

To maximize the effectiveness of rhEPO prescription, it is vital that clinicians carefully select patients for rhEPO therapy. This includes consideration not only of the likely clinical benefits, but also of the likelihood of a hemoglobin increase. In practice, this means paying particular attention to the identification and elimination of other potential causes of anemia (Table 1), and to the identification and treatment of iron deficiency. These activities should precede the prescription of rhEPO, when possible. Figure 1 outlines the current recommendations for patient selection and implementation of rhEPO therapy.

AREAS FOR FURTHER STUDY

In the course of this review, a number of areas for further study have been identified, based on the lack in the current literature of evidence of sufficient quality to aid clinical decision-making. Despite all the studies that have been done, there are no quality data that can unequivocally prove that rhEPO is cost-effective for more than a small number of hemodialysis patients. The Canadian multicenter study (9)—on which the best evidence for the cost-effectiveness of rhEPO is based (38)—excluded diabetic and elderly patients as well as patients who had serious comorbid illness. When attempts have been made to characterize the QOL benefits in more hemodialysis patients, the extent of the QOL benefits is less (55). Presumably the cost-effectiveness of such patients is also more marginal. This issue needs to be addressed urgently for all ESRD populations. As fiscal pressures on government payers mount, there is a real need to have objective data concerning cost-effectiveness of rhEPO in order to maintain even the current modest levels of anemia correction. If the present debate regarding the most appropriate level of hemoglobin for rhEPO-treated patients suggests that a more "normal" hemoglobin

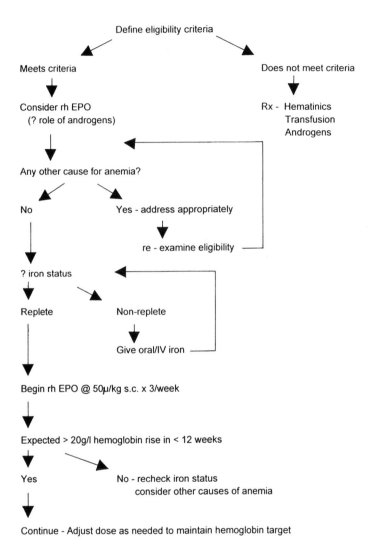

Figure 1   Algorithm for rhEPO administration.

level is desirable, it will be even more important to have supporting data concerning cost-effectiveness.

Perhaps even more important than the cost of raising hematocrit is the currently unknown added potential for adverse effects, particularly hemodialysis access failure and hypertension. At least two large-scale studies are currently under way that are intended to determine the risk–benefit ratio of raising hematocrit. Realistically, no data can be expected from these trials for at least 2 years. In the meantime, physicians are permitting hemoglobins to drift upward, with no clear understanding of the potential consequences—good or bad—for patients.

The suggestion that hematocrit may influence the outcome of renal transplantation is one for which there are few data to make a decision one way or the other. It is, however, a critical issue. The number of cadaveric transplants has been in decline in recent years, at least in some countries (3). Any controllable factor that adversely affects outcome is thus of even more importance than previously. Similarly, the concern that renal function may decline more rapidly in transplant patients given rhEPO for anemia (47) requires closer scrutiny in a larger, prospective trial. As with the predialysis patient population, studies in this area have been too small or of too short a duration, given the slow rate of progress of most progressive renal disease, to provide definitive answers.

Over the past 10 years, a great deal has been learned about the potential of rhEPO to improve the lot of patients with anemia related to ESRD. However, a great deal remains to be learned about how physicians can make the best use of this therapy by developing strategies to bring it to all those who stand to benefit.

REFERENCES

1. Valderrabano F, Jones EHP, Mallick NP. Report on management of renal failure in Europe, XXIV, 1993. Nephrol Dialysis Transplant 1995; 19(suppl 5):S1–S25.
2. USRDS 1994 Annual Report. Am J Kidney Dis 1994; 24(suppl 1):S48–S75.
3. Canadian Organ Replacement Register, 1993. Annual Report, Canadian Institute for Health Information, Don Mills, Ontario, March 1995.
4. Eschbach JW, Adamson JW. Modern aspects of the pathophysiology of renal anemia. Contrib Nephrol 1988; 66:63–70.

5. Winearls CG, Oliver DO, Pippard MJ, Reid C, Downing MR, Cotes PM. Effect of human erythropoietin derived from recombinant DNA on the anaemia of patients maintained by haemodialysis. Lancet 1986; ii:1175– 1177.
6. Eschbach JW, Egrie JC, Downing MR, Browne JK, Adamson JW. Correction of the anemia of end-stage renal disease with recombinant human erythropoietin. N Engl J Med 1987; 316:73–78.
7. Sundal E, Kaeser U. Correction of anaemia of chronic renal failure with recombinant human erythropoietin: safety and efficacy of one year's treatment in a European Multicentre Study of 150 haemodialysis dependent patients. Nephrol Dialysis Transplant 1989; 4:979–987.
8. Eschbach JW, Abdulhadi MH, Browne JK, Delano BG, Downing MR, Egrie JC, Evans RW, Friedman EA, Graber SE, Haley NR. Recombinant human erythropoietin in anemic patients with end-stage renal disease: results of a phase III multicenter trial. Ann Intern Med 1989; 111:992–1000.
9. Canadian Erythropoietin Study Group. Association between recombinant erythropoietin and quality of life and exercise capacity of patients receiving haemodialysis. Br Med J 1990; 300:573–578.
10. Grimm G, Stockenhuber F, Schneeweiss B, Madl C, Zeithofer J, Schneider B. Improvement of brain function in hemodialysis patients treated with erythropoietin. Kidney Int 1990; 38:480–486.
11. Bommer J, Kugel M, Schwobel B, Ritz E, Barth HP, Seelig R. Improved sexual function during recombinant human erythropoietin therapy. Nephrol Dialysis Transplant 1990; 5:204–207.
12. Foley RN, Parfrey PS, Harnett JD, Kent G, Martin CJ, Murray D, Barre PE. Clinical and echocardiographic cardiovascular disease in patients starting end-stage renal disease therapy: prevalence, association and prognosis. Kidney Int 1995; 47:186–192.
13. Silberberg J, Racine, Barre PE, Sniderman AD. Regression of left ventricular hypertrophy in dialysis patients following correction of anemia with recombinant human erythropoietin. Can J Cardiol 1990; 6:1–4.
14. Neff MS, Goldberg J, Slifkin RF, Eiser AR, Colamia V, Kaplan M, Baez A, Gupta S, Mattoo N. A comparison of androgens for anemia in patients on hemodialysis. N Engl J Med 1981; 304:871–875.
15. Cattran DC, Fenton SS, Wilson DR, Oreopoulos D, Shimizu A, Richardson RM. A controlled trial of nandrolone decanoate in the treatment of renal anemia. Kidney Int 1977; 12:430–437.
16. Terasaki PI, Cicciarelli J. Sensitization and its role in transplantation. In: Cerrili GJ, ed. Organ Transplantation and Replacement. New York: Lippincott, 1988:196–207.

17. Walker RH. Special report: transfusion risks. Am J Clin Pathol 1987; 88:374–378.
18. Eschbach JW. Erythropoietin: the promise and the facts. Kidney Int 19??; 45(suppl 44):570–576.
19. Meyer BR. Biotechnology and therapeutics—expensive treatments and limited resources: a view from the hospital. Clin Pharm Ther 1992; 51:359–365.
20. Rosenberg W, Donald A. Evidence based medicine: an approach to clinical problem-solving. Br Med J 1995; 310:1085–1086.
21. Rosenberg W, Donald A. Evidence based medicine: an approach to clinical problem-solving. Br Med J 1995; 310:1085–1086.
22. Carruthers SG, Larochelle P, Haynes RB, Petrasovits A, Schriffin EL. Clinical practice guidelines: report of the Canadian Hypertension Society Consensus Conference. 1. Introduction. Can Med Assoc J 1993; 149:289–292.
23. The U.S. Recombinant Human Erythropoietin Predialysis Study Group. Double-blind, placebo-controlled study of the therapeutic use of recombinant human erythropoietin for anemia associated with chronic renal failure in predialysis patients. Am J Kidney Dis 1991; 18:50–59.
24. Austrian Multicenter Study Group of r-HuEPO in predialysis patients: effectiveness and safety of recombinant human erythropoietin in predialysis patients. Nephron 1992; 61:399–403.
25. Lim VS, DeGowin RL, Zavala D, Kirchner PT, Abels R, Perry P, Fangman J. Recombinant human erythropoietin treatment in pre-dialysis patients: a double blind, placebo-controlled trial. Ann Intern Med 1989; 110:108–114.
26. Frenken LAM, Verberckmoes R, Michielson P, Koene RAP. Efficacy and tolerance of treatment with recombinant human erythropoietin in chronic renal failure (predialysis) patients. Nephrol Dialysis Transplant 1989; 4:782–786.
27. Morris KP, Sharp J, Watson S, Coulthard MG. Non-cardiac benefits of human recombinant erythropoietin in end-stage renal failure and anemia. Arch Dis Child 1993; 69:580–586.
28. Clyne N, Jogestrand T. Effect of erythropoietin treatment on physical exercise capacity and on renal function in predialysis uremic patients. Nephron 1992; 60:390–396.
29. Muirhead N, Goldstein M, Wong C, Steenhuis RE. Correction of anemia in pre-dialysis patients with recombinant human erythropoietin. Am J Kidney Dis. Submitted.

30. Muirhead N, Laupacis A, Wong C. Erythropoietin for anemia in haemodialysis patients: results of a maintenance study (the Canadian Erythropoietin Study Group). Nephrol Dialysis Transplant 1992; 7: 811–816.
31. Klinkmann H, Wieczorek L, Scigalla P. Adverse events of subcutaneous recombinant human erythropoietin: results of a controlled multicentre study. Artif Organs 1993; 17:219–225.
32. Raine AE. Seizures and hypertension events. Sem Nephrol 1990; 10: 40–50.
33. Cassati S, Passerini P, Campise MR, Graziani G, Cesara P, Perisic M, Ponticelli C. Benefits and risks of protracted treatment with human recombinant erythropoietin in patients having haemodialysis. Br Med J 1987; 295:1017–1020.
34. Paganini ED, Lathaur D, Abdulhadi M. Practical considerations of recombinant human erythropoietin therapy. Am J Kidney Dis 1989; 14: 19–28.
35. Churchill DN, Muirhead N, Goldstein M, Posen G, Fay W, Beecroft ML, Gorman J, Taylor DW. Probability of thrombosis of vascular access among hemodialysis patients treated with recombinant human erythropoietin. J Am Soc Nephrol 1994; 4:1809–1813.
36. Tang IY, Vranhos D, Valaitis D, Lau AH. Vascular access thrombosis during recombinant human erythropoietin therapy. ASAIO Trans 1994; 38:M528–M531.
37. McMahon LP, Dawborn JK. Subjective quality of life assessment in hemodialysis patients at different levels of hemoglobin following use of recombinant human erythropoietin. Am J Nephrol 1992; 12:162–169.
38. Sheingold S, Churchill D, Muirhead N, Laupacis A, Labelle R, Goeree R. The impact of recombinant human erythropoietin on medical care costs for hemodialysis patients in Canada. Soc Sci Med 1992; 34:983–991.
39. Stevens ME, Summerfield GP, Hall AA, Beck CA, Harding AJ, Cove-Smith JR, Paterson AD. Cost benefits of low dose subcutaneous erythropoietin in patients with anemia end-stage renal disease. Br Med J 1992; 304:474–477.
40. Besarab A, Flaharty KK, Erslev AJ, McCrea JB, Vlasser PH, Medina F, Caro J, Morris E. Clinical pharmacology and economics of recombinant human erythropoietin in end-stage renal disease: the case for subcutaneous administration. J Am Soc Nephrol 1992; 2:1405–14016.

41. Nissenson AR, Korbet S, Faber M, Burkhart J, Gentile D, Hamburger R, Mattern W, Schreiber M, Swartz R, VanStone J, Watson A, Zimmerman S. Multicenter trial of erythropoietin in patients on peritoneal dialysis. J Am Soc Nephrol 1995; 5:1517–1529.

42. Stevens JM, Auer J, Strong CA, Hughes RT, Oliver DO, Winearls CG, Cotes PM. Stepwise correction of anaemia by subcutaneous administration of human recombinant erythropoietin in patients with chronic renal failure maintained by continuous ambulatory peritoneal dialysis. Nephrol Dialysis Transplant 1991; 6:487–494.

43. Temple RM, Fletcher LF, Deary IJ, Winney RJ. Improved cognitive function in CAPD patients treated with subcutaneous erythropoietin. Nephrol Dialysis Transplant 1991; 6:223–224.

44. Balaskas EV, Melamed IR, Gupta A, Bargman J, Oreopoulos DG. Effect of erythropoietin treatment on nutritional status of continuous ambulatory peritoneal dialysis patients. Perit Dialysis Int 1993; 13: S544–S549.

45. Barany P, Ahberg M, Pettersson E, Tranaeus A, Hultman E, Bergstrom J. Effect of anemia correction with erythropoietin (EPO) on nutritional parameters in continuous peritoneal dialysis (PD) and hemodialysis (HD) patients. Perit Dialysis Int 1992; 12:S98.

46. Jindal KK, Hirsch DJ, Belitsky P, Whalen MA. Low-dose subcutaneous erythropoietin corrects the anemia of renal transplant failure. Nephrol Dialysis Transplant 1992; 7:143–146.

47. Muirhead N, Cattran DC, Zaltzman J, Jindal K, First M, Boucher A, Keown PA, Munch LC. Safety and efficacy of recombinant human erythropoietin in correcting the anemia of patients with chronic renal allograft dysfunction. J Am Soc Nephrol 1994; 5:1216–1222.

48. Grimm PC, Sekiya NM, Robertson LS, Robinson BJ, Ettenger RB. Recombinant human erythropoietin decreases anti-HLA sensitization and may improve renal allograft outcome: involvement of anti-idiotype antibody. Transplant Proc 1991; 23:407–408.

49. Deierhoi MH, Barger BO, Hudson SL, Shroyer TW, Diethelm AG. The effect of erythropoietin and blood transfusions in highly sensitized patients on a single cadaver renal allograft waiting list. Transplantation 1992; 53:363–368.

50. Schmidt R, Kupin W, Dumler F, Venkatt KK, Mozes M. Influence of the pretransplant hematocrit on early graft function in primary cadaveric renal transplantation. Transplantation 1993; 55:1034–1040.

51. Linde T, Wahlberg J, Wikstrom B, Danielson BG. Outcome of renal transplantation in patients treated with erythropoietin. Clin Nephrol 1992; 37:260–263.
52. Ettenger RB, Marik J, Grimm P. The impact of recombinant human erythropoietin therapy on renal transplantation. Am J Kidney Dis 1991; 18:57–61.
53. Eschbach JW, Glenny R, Robertson T, Guthrie M, Rader B, Evans R, Chandler W, Davidson R, Easterling T, Denney J, Schneider G. Normalizing the hematocrit (HCT) in hemodialysis patients with EPO improves quality of life and is safe. J Am Soc Nephrol 1993; 4:425.
54. Powe NR, Griffiths RI, de Lissovoy G, Anderson GF, Watson AJ, Greer JW, Herbert RJ, Eggers PW, Milan RA, Whelton PK. Access to recombinant erythropoietin by medicare: entitled patients in the first year after FDA approval. JAMA 1992; 268:1434–1440.
55. Muirhead N, Churchill DN, Goldstein M, Nadler SP, Posen G, Wong C, Slaughter D, Laplante P. Comparison of subcutaneous and intravenous recombinant erythropoietin for anemia in hemodialysis patients with significant comorbid disease. Am J Nephrol 1992; 12:303–310.
56. Tomson CV, Feehally J, Walls J. Crossover comparison of intravenous and subcutaneous erythropoietin in hemodialysis patients. Nephrol Dialysis Transplant 1992; 7:129–132.
57. Eidemak I, Friedberg MO, Ladefoged SD, Lokkegaard H, Pederson E, Skielboe M. Intravenous versus subcutaneous administration of recombinant human erythropoietin in patients on hemodialysis and CAPD. Nephrol Dialysis Transplant 1992; 7:526–529.
58. Bargman JM, Jones JE, Petro JM. The pharmacokinetics of intraperitoneal erythropoietin administered undiluted or diluted in dialysate. Perit Dialysis Int 1992; 12:369–372.
59. Muirhead N, Keown PA, Slaughter D, Hodsman AB, Cordy PE, Clark WF, Jevnikar AM, Lindsay RM, Fay WP, Hollomby DJ, Wong C, Laupacis A. A double-blind, randomized, dose-finding study of recombinant human erythropoietin in the anaemia of chronic renal failure. Nephrol Dialysis Transplant 1989; 4:477.
60. Granolleras C, Branger B, Shaldon S, Nonnast-Daniel B, Koch KM, Polloh M, Baldamus CA. Subcutaneous erythropoietin: a comparison of daily and thrice weekly administration. Contrib Nephrol 1991; 88: 144–148.
61. Nomoto Y, Kawaguchi Y, Kubota M, Tagawa H, Kubo K, Ogara Y, Shaji T, Kawada Y, Koshikawa S, Mimura N. A multicenter study with once a week or once every two weeks high-dose subcutaneous admini-

stration of recombinant human erythropoietin in continuous ambulatory peritoneal dialysis. Perit Dial Int 1994; 14:56–60.

62. Canadian Erythropoietin Study Group. Effect of recombinant human erythropoietin therapy on blood pressure in hemodialysis patients. Am J Nephrol 1991; 11:23–26.

63. Powe NR, Griffiths RI, Watson AJ, Anderson GF, deLissovoy G, Greer JW, Herbert RJ, Milam RA, Whelton PK. Effect of recombinant erythropoietin on hospital admissions, readmissions, length of stay, and costs of dialysis patients. J Am Soc Nephrol 1994; 4:1455–1465.

64. Churchill DN, Taylor W, Cook RJ, Laplante P, Barre P, Cartier P, Fay WP, Goldstein MB, Jindal K, Mandin H, McKenzie JK, Muirhead N, Parfrey PS, Posen GA, Slaughter D, Ulan RA, Werb R. Canadian hemodialysis morbidity study. Am J Kidney Dis 1992; 19:214–234.

65. Schwab S, Raymond JR, Saeed M, Newman GE, Dennis PA, Bollinger RR. Prevention of hemodialysis fistula thrombosis: early detection of venous stenosis. Kidney Int 1989; 36:707–711.

66. Domoto DT, Bauman JE, Joist JM. Combined aspirin and sulfinpyrazone in the prevention of recurrent hemodialysis vascular access thrombosis. Thromb Res 1991; 62:737–743.

67. Shinaberger JH, Muller JH, Gordner PW. Erythropoietin alert: risks of high hematocrit dialysis. ASAIO Trans 1988; 34:179–184.

68. Zehnder C, Zuber M, Sulzer M, Meyer B, Straumann E, Jenzer HR, Blumberg A. Influence of long-term amelioration of anemia and blood pressure control on left ventricular hypertrophy in hemodialyzed patients. Nephron 1992; 61:21–25.

69. Low-Friedrich I, Grutzmacher P, Marz W, Bergmann M, Schoeppe W. Therapy with recombinant human erythropoietin reduces cardiac size and improves heart function in chronic hemodialysis patients. Am J Nephrol 1991; 11:54–60.

70. Cannella G, LaCanna G, Sandrini M, Gaggiotti M, Nordio D, Movilli E, Mombelloni S, Visiolo O, Maiorca R. Reversal of left ventricular hypertrophy following recombinant human erythropoietin treatment of anaemic dialysed uraemic patients. Nephrol Dial Transplant 1991; 6:31–37.

71. Goldberg N, Lundin AP, Delano B, Friedman EA, Stein RA. Changes in left ventricular size, wall thickness, and function in anemic patients treated with recombinant human erythropoietin. Am Heart J 1992: 124:424–427.

72. Macdougall IC, Lewis NP, Saunders MJ, Cochlin DL, Davies ME, Hutton RD, Fox KA, Coles GA, Williams JD. Long-term cardiorespiratory

effects of amelioration of renal anemia by erythropoietin. Lancet 1990; 335:489–493.

73. Martinez-Vea A, Bardaji A, Garcia C, Ridao C, Richart C, Oiiver JA. Long-term myocardial effects of correction of anemia with recombinant human erythropoietin in aged patients on hemodialysis. Am J Kidney Dis 1992; 19:353–357.

74. London GM, Zins B, Pannier B, Naret C, Berthelot JM, Jacquot C, Sofar M, Drueke TB. Vascular changes in hemodialysis patients in response to recombinant human erythropoietin. Kidney Int 1989; 36: 876–882.

75. Pascual J, Teruel JL, Moya JL, Liano F, Jimenez-Mena M, Ortuno J. Regression of left ventricular hypertrophy after partial correction of anemia with erythropoietin in patients on hemodialysis: a prospective study. Clin Nephrol 1991; 35:280–287.

76. Wizemann V, Schaffer R, Kramer W. Follow-up of cardiac changes induced by anemia compensation in normotensive hemodialysis patients with left ventricular hypertrophy. Nephron 1993; 64:202–206.

77. Whittington R, Barradell LB, Benfield P. Epoetin: a pharmacoeconomic review of its use in chronic renal failure and its effect on quality of life. Pharm Econ 1993; 3:45–82.

12

Analysis of Safety Database for Long-Term Epoetin-β Treatment
A Meta-Analysis Covering 3697 Patients

J. Möcks, W. Franke, B. Ehmer, O. Quarder, and P. Scigalla   Boehringer Mannheim GmbH, Mannheim, Germany

INTRODUCTION

Recombinant human erythropoietin (rhEPO) has become a standard therapy for renal anemia in dialysis patients. The clinical benefits and safety profile of epoetin therapy have been well established. A thorough review of all clinical aspects was published recently by Muirhead et al. (1); see also Refs. 2 and 3. There is, however, comparably little knowledge regarding long-term effects and the safety profile in larger patient groups, given the inherent limitations of individual studies with respect to patient numbers and treatment duration. These questions can effectively be addressed in large database analyses.

Epoetin-β for intravenous and subcutaneous administration has been in clinical development by Boehringer Mannheim since 1987 for the indication of renal anemia. By 1994, a total of 22 clinical trials had been conducted for the purposes of investigating safety and efficacy. In these trials, 3697 patients were treated with epoetin-β for a total period corresponding to almost 4000 patient-years. To meet the regulatory requirements of health authorities, a global database of these studies was created and maintained during the clinical development phase for the purposes of assessing the clinical safety. Because of the large patient numbers and long follow-up (3 years and more) involved in this unselected database, we considered it appropriate to conduct a large-scale meta-analysis to investigate clinical safety and mortality. This chapter details some of the findings.

DATABASE AND METHODS

Table 1 lists some of the properties of the database studies. Of the 22 studies, 18 involved adult hemodialysis patients; 16 of these studies were open-label. Two clinical trials employed a control period at the beginning of the study. One early intravenous trial started with an initial 4-week double-blind control period versus placebo, which was followed by 20 weeks of untreated control, after which all patients in the study received epoetin-β. The second controlled trial with subcutaneous epoetin administration lasted 2 years. In the first

Table 1 Overview of the Contents of the Database in Renal Anemia

Clinical development	1987–1994
Clinical studies (total)	22
Patients under epoetin	3697 (3951 patient-years)
Controlled studies (ESRD) (2)	244 vs. 246 patients (200 patient-years)
Predialysis studies (2)	270 patients (170 patient-years)
Studies in children (2)	209 patients (150 patient-years)
CAPD study (1)	107 patients (50 patient-years)
Intravenous administration	2599 patients
Start dose (in 60%)	100–150 U/kg body weight per week
Subcutaneous administration	1093 patients
Start dose (in 67%)	50–100 U/kg body weight per week

year, epoetin patients were compared with untreated controls; in the second, both treatment groups received epoetin. Two studies investigated predialysis patients and two studied involved children. One study dealt with patients on continuous ambulatory peritoneal dialysis (CAPD).

In the database as a whole, the mean age at enrollment was 49.6 years (SD = 18.6). The youngest patient was aged 1 year and the oldest 86 years. Female patients constituted 55% of the treated population; there was a preponderance of female patients in the group of those aged 60 and over (64%). Gender was approximately evenly distributed in all other age groups.

Higher initial doses with i.v. administration were predominantly used in the early phase of the clinical development. Subsequently, the s.c. route of administration, with lower initial doses, predominated. Table 2 summarizes the dosing data.

In some of the trials, the patients were treated for more than 3 years. 1820 patients were treated for longer than one year, while 452 patients and 99 patients receiving epoetin were treated for longer than 2 and 3 years, respectively. Table 3 summarizes the exposure data. Despite the reduction in patient numbers over the 3 years, the database still offers 452 patients at the start of the third year, which is not low compared to many studies and allows for some analyses.

Table 2 Overview of Dosing in Epoetin-β Trials

Doses U/kg/wk	All periods		Initial doses	
	i.v.	s.c.	i.v.	s.c.
1–50	819	765	18	187
51–100	1782	1203	169	732
101–150	2237	775	1616	143
151–250	1559	410	577	22
251–500	811	139	218	8
501–750	94	4	—	1
751–1000	17	—	1	—
1001–1500	2	—	—	—
≥1501	1	—	—	—

Table 3   Overview of Patient Exposure (the exposure period for each patient was extended, where applicable, by up to 6 weeks of observation following the last dose)

| | All routes | |
	Epoetin	Control
≥1 day	3697	246
>2 weeks	3667	244
>5 weeks	3590	240
>13 weeks	3247	228
>26 weeks (0.5 year)	2695	178
>52 weeks (1.0 year)	1820	57
>78 weeks (1.5 years)	882	10
>104 weeks (2.0 years)	452	4
>130 weeks (2.5 years)	163	—
>156 weeks (3.0 years)	99	—
Total patients years	3951	197

In accordance with the state of the art in clinical studies, all adverse events, irrespective of the causal relationship with treatment, were recorded in the studies. The adverse events were defined* and encoded according to international standards. Adverse events cannot be identified with side effects of treatment but describe a much larger class of clinical events.

The principle of recording all adverse events irrespective of a possible relationship with treatment leads to a large number of adverse events resulting from the underlying morbidity of patients in end-stage renal disease. Because of this morbidity, all the patients can be expected to experience at least one adverse event. In practice, however, this figure was 67%. It is one of the primary tasks of a safety

---

*An adverse event is any undesired, noxious, or pathological change in a patient or subject, as indicated by signs, symptoms, and/or laboratory changes, that occurs in association with the use of a drug or placebo whether or not considered drug-related. This definition includes intercurrent illnesses or injuries, exacerbation of preexisting conditions, and adverse events occurring as a result of drug withdrawal, abuse, or overdose.

analysis to identify, in this large pool, those adverse events constituting potential adverse reactions to therapy. Incidences of the various adverse-event categories were determined, and potential factors influencing these incidences were investigated. In addition to a comparison of the controlled conditions, the investigation of these incidences over time and in the various dosage groups is especially important. This particularly applies in situations involving long-term treatment, as is the case with epoetin, during which placebo control cannot be maintained for ethical reasons.

Estimating incidences for the various adverse-event categories requires methods that take into account the fact that patients remained in the studies for differing periods, particularly across multiple studies. Such "failure time" methods count each event at its first onset so as to provide cumulative incidences for each treatment period (methodology of survival analysis). Observations that were terminated before the considered event occurred (so-called censored observations) can be incorporated and still yield a valid estimate. It is important to note that these methods allow for any underlying course of the risk per unit time (hazard) for experiencing the event—in contrast with the simple adjustment to total patient-years, which is meaningful only when the underlying hazard takes a constant course. The reduction in patients treated as the 3 years progress, as reflected in Table 3, will naturally increase the variability and diminish the precision of the estimated figures compared to those obtained in the first year.

The mortality analysis presented below also utilized survival analysis, in which the event was defined on the day of death (rather than the date of onset of the adverse event leading to death). Any death was counted, irrespective of the time since the last epoetin dose. To achieve a more detailed analysis, the chronological development of the risk per unit time (hazard) was estimated nonparametrically by kernel smoothing of the Nelson hazard estimate according to Müller and Wang (4). This approach amounts to a weighted moving average in which the bandwidth of smoothing was adapted over time according to the number of patients treated. The course of the hazard is important for exploratory interpretation: a constant course generally suggests no association of treatment with the underlying risk. If a significant nonconstant course is observed, the period of treatment is assumed to exert some influence on the risk. Constancy was tested statistically by a test described by Hollander and Proschan (5). This goodness-of-fit test is suitable for censored observations. The null distribution (assuming a constant hazard) was obtained by maximum likelihood estimation of the constant (events per total observation time). The test is very conservative under the null hypothesis when the constant is first estimated from the data. Thus, the type I error is much smaller than 5%, for example, when this was the fixed level of significance, if the null hypothesis is in fact true.

The following approach was chosen for analyzing general morbidity in the patients: as most of the adverse events are related to the disease and not to treatment, the percentage of days on which adverse events were experienced represents a measure of general morbidity. The temporal development of this measure over 2 years was for this measure in the controlled s.c. study.

RESULTS

Hypertensive Events

Analyses with reports of hypertensive events are summarized in Figure 1. The upper part displays the incidences over time in half-year periods for up to 3 years of treatment.

In the first year, controlled conditions can also be compared. It is seen that there is a marked time trend toward early increase in the risk to suffer first from a hypertensive event. Incidences in controlled conditions are lower in untreated controls compared to epoetin patients. There is no evidence of any late or cumulative effects of epoetin-β. The concentration of hypertensive events in the early stages suggests that treatment does have an influence on this incidence. A certain amount of reporting bias may also be present (overreporting at the start of a study of an identified side effect), as reflected in the results for the controls.

The analysis was also performed for serious hypertensive events. In accordance with the international definition, these were hyper-

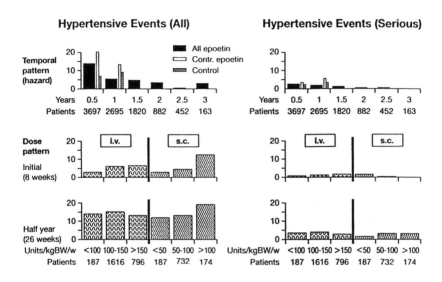

Figure 1 Incidences of hypertensive events over time and in the various dose groups. Patient numbers refer to those starting the respective therapy phase ("all epoetin"). "Contr. epoetin" refers to $n = 244$ patients treated with epoetin in studies in which a parallel untreated control group of $n = 246$ was available ("control").

tensive events that were fatal or life-threatening, resulted in or prolonged hospitalization, or led to significant disability or sequelae. Reporting bias can be neglected out in this case. A temporal trend is not apparent since the incidences plot a flat course over the treatment period. Thus, this analysis did not reveal any influence of epoetin therapy on the occurrence of serious hypertensive events.

The lower part of Figure 1 displays results for dose trends. Due to differing initial dosing, dose groups were separately formed for i.v. and s.c. administration. The upper part shows early results at 8 weeks after start of therapy, while the incidences in the lower part are shown after 6 months (maintenance phase). In the correction phase, both i.v. and s.c. administration routes exhibit a clear dose trend for all hypertensive events (left). In the maintenance phase, the dose trend is still visible for s.c. treatment, but less so for i.v.

treatment. The two lower-dose groups receiving s.c. treatment resulted in the smallest cumulative incidence after 6 months. In interpreting these results, it appears that the overall level of hypertensive risk can be minimized through a slow, gradual (i.e., low-dosage) correction of anemia. No dose trend is discernible for serious hypertensive events, which suggests that epoetin has no effect in this respect.

Thromboembolic Events

Figure 2 displays the database results for thromboembolic events as for hypertensive events. The results for vascular access thromboses are presented on the left. In this case, the number of patients differs because only patients on hemodialysis can experience this adverse event.

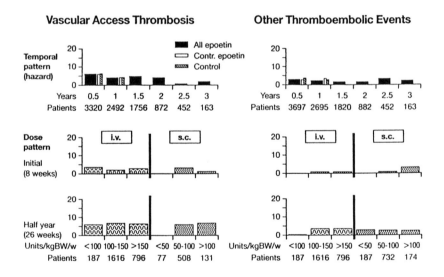

Figure 2 Incidences of thromboembolic events over time and in the various dose groups. Patient numbers refer to those starting the respective therapy phase. Patient numbers for vascular access thrombosis refer to those studies with patients on hemodialysis ("all epoetin"). "Contr. epoetin" refers to $n = 244$ patients treated with epoetin in studies in which a parallel untreated control group of $n = 246$ was available ("control").

There was no marked time trend for incidences over 3 years and no discernible difference in controlled conditions. Nor was any dose trend apparent for either the correction or the maintenance phases. This analysis did not, therefore, provide any indication of an influence of epoetin on this incidence. A distinction cannot be made in the database between native grafts and artificial grafts. For other thromboembolic events, e.g., deep-vein thromboses (right side of figure), no pattern suggestive of any influence of epoetin therapy was seen.

Predialysis

Whether epoetin therapy influenced the progression of predialysis patients to terminal renal failure was investigated in a trial conducted by Koch et al. (6). Figure 3 shows the course of 1/creatinine as a measure of deterioration of renal function for 100 days before and after the onset of epoetin-β therapy. The decline in the measure was

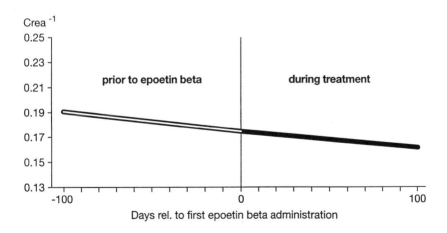

Figure 3   Predialysis patients: development of 1/creatinine before and after the start of epoetin-β therapy. The trace characterizes the mean development for all patients as obtained from individual regression analyses (independently estimated before and after start of treatment).

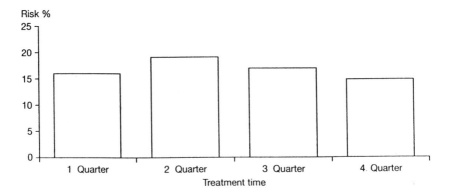

Figure 4   Predialysis patients ($n = 270$): the risk of progression to end-stage renal failure after start of therapy in 3-month intervals.

estimated by linear regression on an individual-patient basis separately for the pre- and posttherapy phases. Figure 3 shows the resulting mean slope. It is clear that the onset of epoetin therapy has no influence on the speed of deterioration of renal function in terms of this parameter. This question was further analyzed by means of the estimated risk of progression to dialysis (which was a clinical endpoint in this study). The results are displayed in Figure 4 for 3-month intervals after therapy onset. The resulting flat profile does not provide any indication of an influence of epoetin-β on the course of this risk.

General Morbidity

In the controlled trial, 181 patients received epoetin for 1 year while 180 patients remained without epoetin during this time. Thereafter, both treatment groups continued on epoetin for a second year. General morbidity of the patients was measured on the basis of the percentage of days with adverse events. The temporal course for this parameter is presented in Figure 5. In the initial phase, patients on epoetin-β were worse than controls in this respect. As therapy progresses, the increase in morbidity flattens off, while the untreated

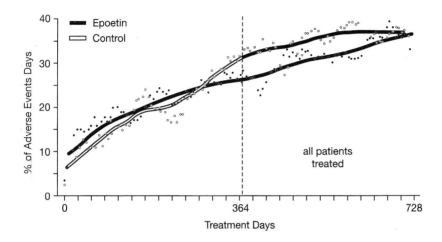

Figure 5 Controlled study (epoetin $n = 181$; control $n = 180$): course of the percentage of days with adverse events over 2 years.

control group maintains a steep, almost linear progression. By the end of 1 year, patients in the epoetin-β group were experiencing fewer days with adverse events than the controls. In the second year, epoetin was initiated for the control group and maintained for 1 further year. This led to a similar reduction in the progression of general morbidity. Both groups approach each other at the end of the second year.

Global Mortality

Mortality data are reliable since no subjective assessment is involved. They represent the most serious possible outcome of an adverse event, and reporting compliance can be assumed in this respect. The results of the first mortality analysis, which concerned all patients in the database, are given in Figure 6. As with other incidences, the mortality results represent conditional risk; i.e., the risk is given relative to the actual cohort starting the respective interval and not as a percentage of the initial cohort.

In the first year of epoetin therapy, mortality is reduced, compared to controls, by about 20%, primarily in relation to the cardio-

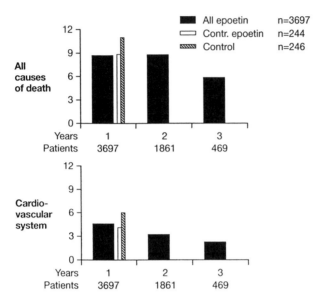

Figure 6 Mortality analysis: annual mortality risk in the total database and for controlled studies. "Contr. epoetin" refers to $n = 244$ patients treated with epoetin in studies in which a parallel untreated control group of $n = 246$ was available ("control").

vascular system (40%). The relative risks assessed by the Cox model were 0.8 and 0.6 for all causes and cardiovascular causes, respectively. Other causes of death involved a relative risk approaching 1. These reductions failed to achieve statistical significance because of an insufficient number of patients. The subsequent course for mortality risk in the total database exhibits a persistent decline, particularly after the second year of treatment, down to an annual risk of about 6%. (The slight difference in patient numbers here from those in, for example, Figure 1 or Table 3, is due to the unrestricted inclusion of postdose follow-up periods, where applicable, in the mortality analysis.) The reduction was seen mainly in cardiovascular deaths.

As these results clearly merit a closer look, the patient group was restricted to the 3111 adult hemodialysis patients in the database. The continuous course of all-cause mortality risk, subdivided

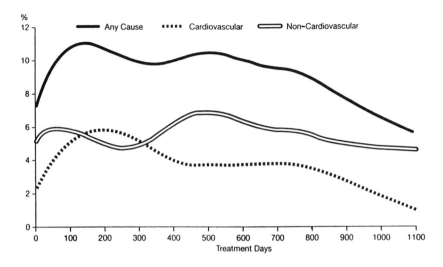

Figure 7 Mortality analysis: adult patients on hemodialysis. Estimated hazard functions over 3 years (scaled in annual risk).

into cardiovascular and other risk, was analyzed by continuous hazard function estimates. The results are given in Figure 7.

All-cause mortality (solid line) increased in the first 100 days from about 8% to over 10%. This effect reflects the fact that, since no moribund patients were included in the clinical trials, the risk reached normal levels only after a certain latency period (a similar rise was seen for control patients). After about 500 days, a steady decline in mortality risk was observed. This reduction was statistically significant according to the test of Hollander and Proschan: $p < 1\%$. The test also resulted in $p < 1\%$ for data restricted to the course after 100 days. This additional test was performed in order to exclude the initial rise in the hazard. The course of cardiovascular mortality (dotted line) closely resembles that for all-cause mortality (tests significant). Other noncardiovascular mortality (double line) exhibits a roughly constant course over the 3 years, which argues against the influence of epoetin on this risk.

The composition of the all-cause mortality risk is analyzed in Figure 8. After an initial rise to about 50% for cardiovascular

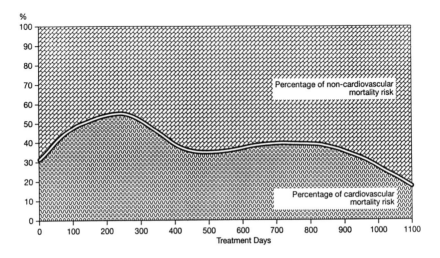

Figure 8 Mortality analysis: adult patients on hemodialysis. Course of the composition of all-cause mortality risk.

mortality as a percentage of all-cause mortality (which is in keeping with usual figures), a decline was observed in the percentage of cardiovascular mortality to about 30% after 2.5 years. This also suggests the occurrence of a change in the composition of all-cause mortality risk during long-term therapy.

Is the decline in mortality risk to about 6% a trustworthy and stable effect of epoetin-β therapy? A number of analyses were conducted to check the sensitivity of the results. There appears to be no selection by age: patients starting the third year of therapy were, on average, just 2 years older than those starting the first year. The influence of study subgroups and patient dropouts on the trend in mortality was checked in several additional analyses. The general trend of a reduction in mortality was verified in all runs. In particular, a possible bias through study dropouts due to adverse events was ruled out by worst-case calculations. Other possible important factors—including initial disease status, e.g., diabetes, and duration and method of dialysis—cannot be investigated at the present time because of the restricted information content in the database.

DISCUSSION

Database analyses deal with data that have already been collected, possibly for other purposes. Consequently, they inherently provide a mainly descriptive and/or exploratory basis for interpretation. While lacking the confirmatory strength of prospective clinical trials, databases nevertheless offer the advantage of large numbers of patients. The present database was built for documenting the clinical safety of epoetin-β and covers all studies (not specifically selected) involved in the clinical development program for renal anemia.

The incidence and course of hypertensive events did not present any surprises. The results of the database compare well with the figures reported in the literature (compare to Ref. 1). Since hypertension is a common problem in uremic patients, it is difficult to differentiate between "spontaneous" hypertension and events induced or aggravated by epoetin. There is no doubt that epoetin induces hypertensive events, but the analysis with serious hypertensive events did not result in data indicating any influence of epoetin on their occurrence. In other words, most of the cases of hypertension induced by epoetin remained mild and manageable. Still, it is recommended that blood pressure be closely monitored, particularly at the start of therapy. Anemia should be corrected slowly and gradually by low initial dosing. The blood pressure in patients at risk of uncontrolled hypertension should, of course, be well under control before treatment begins, and, if necessary, a change in antihypertensive treatment or dialysis regimen should be considered.

It is perhaps surprising that the database analyses did not find any evidence of an adverse effect of epoetin on the incidence of thromboembolic events. However, the database does not allow differentiation between native and artificial grafts in dialysis patients, which was discussed (compare to Ref. 1) as a factor influencing the risk of vascular access thrombosis. The results still suggest that no strong influence, at least, of epoetin exists in these events.

Another question for discussion is whether, as a result of an increase in the viscosity of the blood, epoetin could adversely influence the filtration function of the kidney and thereby accelerate the progression to end-stage disease in predialysis patients. The results of an American study (7) and of the study presented here (6) did not show a steeper decline for 1/creatinine after the start of epoetin compared to the preceding period. Furthermore, the risk of progression to end-stage disease after the start of therapy was not dependent on the treatment duration.

The results of the database relating to general morbidity indicate a positive effect of epoetin-β. The exploratory analysis showed gains for epoetin therapy in reducing the progression of morbidity. This trend underlines a long-term benefit for epoetin therapy, which certainly can also be assumed to achieve gains in general quality of life.

The most important and promising result of the database analysis is the reduction in long-term mortality risk. Mortality represents the ultimate criterion of any therapy and should, at least, not be increased.

The results here show a decrease for this figure to about 6% of annual mortality risk in the third year—a result that deserves further scrutiny. The question arises as to whether other influential factors changed during treatment, or whether some other selective mechanism contributed to the favorable development. Sensitivity analyses showed, for example, that age does not constitute a selection effect, and that the decline in mortality was not biased by patients dropping out from the studies. The patients entering the third year of therapy consist of responders to epoetin-β and the therapy was also well tolerated by these patients. Their general condition was likely to be improved by therapy. Whether some other selective mechanism, or important factors such as quality and duration of dialysis or concomitant disease, e.g., diabetes, had possibly changed and thereby contributed to the positive result cannot be investigated at present, as these data elements do not form part of the present database. Further research is needed to investigate the interaction of these factors with long-term epoetin therapy.

A particularly suggestive outcome of this analysis was the fact that the decline in mortality seems to be exclusively attributable to a decline in cardiovascular deaths. Other risks remained unaffected by the treatment period. This was further underlined by the observed change in the composition of the risk in favor of a lower proportion of cardiovascular risk. The assumption of positive effects of epoetin on cardiovascular factors is certainly not far-fetched (8). Since epoetin improves tissue oxygenation, it may also positively influence cardiac function, coronary artery disease, and left ventricular hypertrophy. These effects have been reported in several studies. Left ventricular hypertrophy, in particular, has been identified as an independent and major factor in cardiovascular mortality risk (9; see also Chapter 6). This background provides further support for a possible contribution of epoetin-β toward a decrease in mortality risk.

REFERENCES

1. Muirhead N, Bargmann J, Burgess E, Kailash KJ, Levin A, Nolin L, Parfrey P. Evidence-based recommendations for the clinical use of recombinant human erythropoietin. Am J Kidney Dis 1995; 26:1–24.
2. Dunn CJ, Wagstaff AJ. Epoetin alfa: a review of its clinical efficacy in the management of anaemia associated with renal failure and chronic disease and its use in surgical patients. Drug Aging 1995; 2:131–156.
3. Patterson KG. The uses of recombined human erythropoietin. Saudi Med J 1994; 15(1):1–13.
4. Müller HG, Wang JL. Hazard rate estimation under random censoring with varying kernels and bandwidths. Biometrics 1994; 50:61–75.
5. Hollander M, Proschan F. Testing to determine the underlying distribution using randomly censored data. Biometrics 1979; 35:393–401.
6. Koch KM, Koene RAP, Messinger D, Quarder O, Scigalla P. The use of epoetin beta in anemic predialysis patients with chronic renal failure. Clin Nephrol 1995; 40:201–208.
7. The US Recombinant Human Erythropoietin Predialysis Study Group. Double-blind, placebo-controlled study of the therapeutic use of recombinant human erythropoietin for anemia associated with chronic renal failure in predialysis patients. Am J Kidney Dis 1991; 18:50–59.
8. Ritz E, Zeier M, Schneider P, Jones E. Cardiovascular mortality of patients with polycystic kidney on dialysis: is there a lesson to learn? Nephron 1994; 66:125–128.
9. Silberberg JS, Barre PE, Prichard JS, Sniderman AD. Impact of left ventricular hypertrophy on survival in end-stage renal disease. Kidney Int 1989; 36:286–290.

13

Iron Therapy
Overview and Recommendations

Iain C. Macdougall King's College and Dulwich Hospitals, London, England

INTRODUCTION

When recombinant human erythropoietin (EPO) was launched onto the European market around 1990, the development of functional iron deficiency and the need for iron supplementation were scarcely anticipated. Indeed, the magnitude of this problem associated with EPO therapy took the nephrological world by surprise. We are now aware that an inadequate iron supply to the bone marrow is the most common cause of an impaired response to EPO, and that this deficiency is best treated with intravenous iron supplementation (1–3). We have come to realize that oral iron replacement often does not keep pace with the requirements of the marrow for iron, but are still unsure of the best methods for detecting functional iron deficiency (3). In addition, there are no universally recognized regimens for the administration of i.v. iron, and different countries in the world have access to different iron preparations.

The aim of this chapter is to review the current status of iron therapy associated with EPO: why dialysis patients are prone to develop iron deficiency, how best to monitor this condition, and how best to treat it. Many questions remain unanswered, but it is hoped that ongoing interest and research in this important aspect of EPO management will yield new information and solutions to these unresolved issues.

WHY ARE DIALYSIS PATIENTS PRONE TO DEVELOP IRON DEFICIENCY?

Even prior to the advent of EPO therapy, many patients with end-stage renal failure had a tendency to develop iron deficiency. This was usually an *absolute* iron deficiency, characterized by exhaustion of total body iron stores and manifested by low serum ferritin levels. This condition results from a state of negative iron balance developing over many months or years and exacerbated by a number of factors. Normal iron balance in nonuremic individuals is usually achieved by the inevitable gastrointestinal losses of iron—amounting to approximately 1 mg a day—being offset by a similar dietary intake. Patients with end-stage renal failure generally have a higher than normal degree of occult gastrointestinal blood loss (4,5), amounting to as much as 4–5 mg a day, due to an increased incidence of gastroesophagitis and peptic ulceration (6), along with an enhanced bleeding tendency due to uremic platelet dysfunction (7). This may also be exacerbated in hemodialysis patients by intermittent heparin administration given during the dialysis session and by the frequent therapeutic use of aspirin. The procedure of hemodialysis also results in significant losses of blood (and hence iron) in the dialyser and dialysis lines (8). Renal failure patients are subjected to frequent venipuncture for blood tests, and amounts of between 2 and 6 liters of blood loss a year have been estimated. Some female dialysis patients may also suffer from menorrhagia. Furthermore, these excessive losses often occur in association with reduced oral iron intake, due to either poor dietary intake as a result of anorexia or impaired iron absorption from the gut exacerbated by concomitant use of other medications such as phosphate binders. Although many studies in the 1970s showed that dialysis patients with iron deficiency absorb oral iron effectively (9–12), this is not universally the case, and there are certainly some patients who have poor absorption of iron from the gut.

It is into this scenario that EPO was introduced 6 or 7 years ago. In addition to the stresses causing negative iron balance just described, patients treated with EPO are expected to have increases in hemoglobin concentration of around 5 g/dl (from 6–7 g/dl up to 11–12 g/dl). Manufacture of red cells equivalent to this rise in hemoglobin requires a large quantity of iron (equivalent to a serum ferritin of at least 100 μg/L) (13). It is therefore not altogether surprising that many patients given EPO exhaust what borderline stores of iron they have, and develop *absolute* iron deficiency. What was not anticipated was the widespread development of *functional* iron deficiency (3). Patients with more than adequate levels of total body iron stores (as indicated by normal or high serum ferritin levels) began showing impaired responses to EPO therapy as a result of a failure to mobilize iron from its stores in the reticuloendothelial system and deliver it to the marrow for erythropoiesis (Figure 1). The first published report of functional iron deficiency associated with EPO therapy appeared in the *New England Journal of Medicine* paper by Eschbach et al. in 1987 (14). This patient had an initial response to EPO but after 10–12 weeks this tailed off, corresponding with a decrease in transferrin saturation from 51 to 13% although the serum ferritin was well-maintained at 578 μg/L. Administration of i.v. iron dextran restored both the hemoglobin and reticulocyte responses (Figure 2). Subsequent studies have confirmed the high incidence of functional iron deficiency in dialysis patients receiving EPO therapy (3).

MONITORING OF IRON STATUS IN PATIENTS RECEIVING EPO

To determine which patients require additional iron supplementation, it is important to be able to detect reliably the development of iron deficiency (either absolute or functional). Unfortunately no single test exists that is absolutely ideal for this purpose, partly because

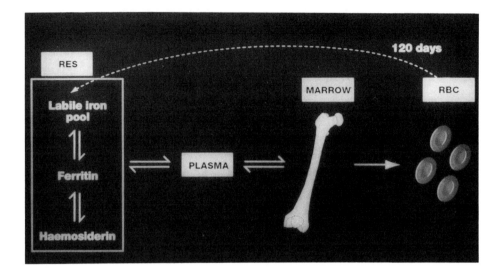

Figure 1   Schematic representation of iron metabolism. RES = reticuloendothelial system.

of the complex nature of the processes involved in iron metabolism (Figure 1). A number of tests are available, however (Table 1), that have varying usefulness in monitoring iron status in patients receiving EPO (3).

The *serum ferritin* is an indirect measure of the total body iron stores, and in normal individuals a level of less than $15 \mu g/L$ indicates *absolute* iron deficiency. In renal failure, however, the relationship between serum ferritin and iron stores is not as precise, and different threshold values of serum ferritin as an indicator of iron deficiency have been suggested, such as $50 \mu g/L$ (12), $70 \mu g/L$ (15), and $80 \mu g/L$ (16). Second, a normal or high serum ferritin level does not exclude functional iron deficiency, as discussed earlier. Thus, the serum ferritin may suggest adequate or even excessive iron stores but gives no indication of how easily this iron can be released and made available to the marrow for hemoglobin synthesis. Third, the serum ferritin level may be surprisingly raised in inflammatory conditions, infec-

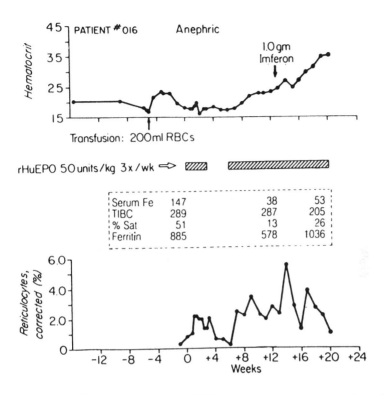

Figure 2 Sluggish response to EPO corrected by administration of i.v. iron dextran despite adequate serum ferritin levels. (From Ref. 14.)

Table 1 Tests for Detecting Iron Deficiency

Serum tests
    Serum ferritin
    Serum iron
    Serum total iron binding capacity (TIBC)
    Transferrin saturation
    Serum transferrin receptor
Red cell tests
    MCV, MCH, MCHC
    Hypochromic red cells
    Red cell ferritin
    Free erythrocyte protoporphyrin
    Red cell zinc protoporphyrin
Other tests
    Marrow stainable iron
    Ferrokinetic studies

185

tion, and liver disease (17,18). Despite these limitations, this marker of iron status is the most widely used test to monitor patients on EPO, and it is the best available guide to the adequacy of iron stores at the start of treatment. Thus, patients with initial ferritin levels less than 100 μg/L will almost certainly require i.v. iron supplementation to support the requirements of the marrow during active erythropoiesis (2,19).

In theory, the *transferrin saturation* should be a better indicator of how much iron is available to the bone marrow for erythropoiesis since it reflects the circulating amount of iron in the plasma relative to the total iron-binding capacity (20). Previous studies suggested that once the transferrin saturation level falls below 16%, the iron supply for erythropoiesis will be inadequate (21). The main problem with this measurement, however, is that it shows a marked diurnal variation, which is due to wide fluctuations in plasma iron concentration and is not related to the assay used (13). Furthermore, the assay is laborious and time-consuming, and the reliability of the measurement is also dependent on which method is used.

Measurement of the percentage of *hypochromic red cells* is probably the best indicator of functional iron deficiency at the present time (Figure 3) (3,22). This method measures, on the full blood count sample, the proportion of red cells in circulation that have an individual cell hemoglobin concentration less than 28 g/dl. In normal individuals this is usually less than 2.5%, and in renal patients receiving EPO, values greater than 10% are strongly suggestive of functional iron deficiency. This method is simple, rapid, and inexpensive, but it does require access to a Technicon H1, H2, or H3 automated cell counter which uses a flow cytometric method for analysis. Unfortunately, not every center has the use of one of these instruments; thus, this method is limited by its availability.

Other markers of iron deficiency either have not been adequately assessed in patients on EPO therapy or, again, are not widely available. Measurement of the *red cell ferritin* is probably more sensitive in reflecting iron needs than the serum ferritin, and is less affected by inflammatory conditions or liver disease (23). *Red cell zinc protoporphyrin* levels are elevated in iron deficiency and lead poisoning, but the presence of uremic metabolites and drugs may interfere

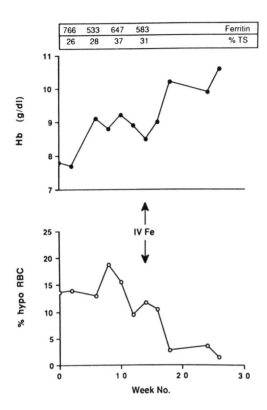

766	533	647	583		Ferritin
26	28	37	31		% TS

Figure 3 Use of percentage hypochromic red cells to detect functional iron deficiency in a dialysis patient receiving EPO.

with the assay and give spurious results (24). *Serum transferrin receptor levels* correlate well with the degree of erythropoietic activity, and levels will also be raised in iron deficiency (25); this test, however, is useful as a marker of iron deficiency only in steady-state erythropoiesis and its value in patients receiving EPO is therefore limited.

WHAT IS THE OPTIMAL REGIMEN FOR GIVING IRON SUPPLEMENTATION?

Assuming that one has proven, or suspects, iron deficiency (e.g., ferritin <100 μg/L, transferrin saturation <20%, or hypochromic red

Table 2   Iron Preparations Available Worldwide

Oral
    Ferrous sulfate
    Ferrous fumarate
    Ferrous gluconate
    Ferrous succinate
    Ferrous glycine sulfate
    Iron polymaltose

Intravenous
    Iron dextran
    Iron hydroxysaccharate (sucrose)
    Iron dextrin (polymaltose)
    Iron sodium gluconate
    Iron sorbitol citrate

cells >10%), what is the best way to replace the iron deficit? Three routes of iron administration are available (oral, intramuscular, and intravenous), and there are many different preparations on the market (Table 2). *Oral* administration has the benefit of simplicity and is very cheap. Side effects, however, are common, particularly gastrointestinal intolerance causing anorexia, nausea, vomiting, abdominal pain, constipation, and diarrhea; this frequently results in poor compliance. These side effects are dose-related and hence are more common in the preparations that contain larger amounts of elemental iron. One preparation has few advantages over another, and ferrous sulfate is as good as any. The iron is more readily absorbed if not taken with food, but side effects are then more common. If nausea is a problem, then it is best to recommend taking the iron tablets with meals, but absorption is then less good. Iron tablets should not be taken along with phosphate binders because, again, the latter will interfere with absorption.

    Unfortunately, it has become very apparent that oral iron administration is frequently not able to keep pace with iron requirements in patients receiving EPO (3). This may be due partly to poor compliance, but due mainly to the fact that impaired absorption from the gut limits the amount of iron able to reach the marrow. Because of this, and the economic consequences of wasting EPO in a patient responding poorly because of iron deficiency, there has been an increasing trend to use i.v. iron. This is much preferred to the *intramuscular* route, which should be avoided in this clinical setting for several reasons: the injection is painful; it causes persistent brownish discoloration of the skin; absorption and bioavailability from this route are highly variable; muscle sarcomas have been reported; and bleeding into the muscle may occur, particularly since these patients already have an increased bleeding tendency due to uremia.

A number of *intravenous* iron preparations are available worldwide, but the choice is limited by the country of origin. Thus, iron dextran is used widely in the United States and Canada, where it is the only preparation available; iron hydroxysaccharate (sucrose) is used extensively in Sweden, Germany, and Austria; iron dextrin (polymaltose) is widely used in France; and iron sodium gluconate is used in a number of European countries, including Germany.

ARE ALL I.V. IRON PREPARATIONS THE SAME?

The answer is most definitely no; there are major differences in the molecular size of the various iron complexes, and in their degradation kinetics, their iron availability characteristics, and their side-effect profiles (Table 3). In general, the larger the iron complex molecule, the more tightly the iron is bound. This results in slower degradation kinetics and iron release, but also an enhanced safety profile; thus, larger doses can be given more safely (e.g., iron dextran). At the opposite end of the spectrum are iron complex preparations of low molecular weight such as iron sodium gluconate. These release iron very readily, and there is a danger of free iron dissociating in circulation if too high doses are used. There is also a risk of parenchymal liver damage if excessive doses are given, since some of the iron preparation may be taken up by the hepatocytes in addition to the reticuloendothelial system (RES) (26). With the greater-molecular-weight complexes such as iron dextran, virtually all the iron is taken

Table 3 Comparison of I.V. Iron Preparations

Type	Examples of preparations	Characteristics	Molecular weight	Degradation kinetics constant $(k \times 10^3/min)$	Uptake by hepatocytes	Side effects
I	Iron dextran; iron dextrin (polymaltose)	Robust/strong	>100,000	15–50	No	Anaphylactic reactions with iron dextran; serum sickness (fever, myalgia, arthralgia); may worsen rheumatoid arthritis
II	Iron hydroxy-saccharate (sucrose)	Semirobust/medium strong	30,000–100,000	50–100	No	Metallic taste; hypotension (if injected too quickly); arthralgia (high doses)
III	Iron sodium gluconate; iron sorbitol citrate	Labile/weak	<50,000	>100	Possibly	Hypotension; loin pain; epigastric pain
IV	Jectofer (iron citrate, iron sorbitol, iron dextrin); Ferrlicit (iron gluconate, iron dextrin)	Mixtures containing at least two different iron complexes			Depends on individual constituents	Gastrointestinal side effects; metallic taste; myalgia; possible severe circulatory failure/hypotension

up by the RES, even at high doses. Most of these data, however, have been obtained from animal toxicity studies (26) and should be interpreted as such.

Thus, from a practical point of view, all the i.v. iron preparations provide readily available iron for erythropoiesis. Iron sodium gluconate has a less favorable side-effect profile and should be used in small doses (maximum 62.5–125 mg). Iron dextran may be safely given up to a dose of 1000 mg but carries an appreciable risk of anaphylactic reactions due to naturally occurring circulating dextran antibodies. Iron hydroxysaccharate can be given up to a dose of 200 mg and probably offers the best compromise in terms of iron availability and safety.

WHAT IS THE BEST REGIMEN FOR ADMINISTERING I.V. IRON?

The regimen used for giving i.v. iron will depend on:

1. *The availability of the i.v. iron preparation.* As discussed above, most countries have access to only one or two preparations.
2. *The dialysis modality of the patient.* It is quite feasible to administer small doses of i.v. iron with each dialysis session three times a week in a hospital-based hemodialysis patient; this is clearly impractical in a CAPD patient, in whom larger, less frequent doses should be given.
3. *The iron preparation used.* As discussed above, iron sodium gluconate is best given in small repeated doses, whereas larger doses of iron hydroxysaccharate and iron dextran may be given.
4. *The likelihood of side effects.* Larger doses of i.v. iron are more likely to precipitate hypotension, myalgia, and arthralgia, whereas smaller doses are better tolerated. Patients who have a history of multiple allergies or atopy should also avoid iron dextran, if possible, in view of the increased risk of anaphylaxis.

5. *Personal clinician preference.*   Most nephrologists agree that in CAPD or predialysis patients it is impractical to give i.v. iron more than once a month, and hence an infusion of 200–1000 mg over 30–60 minutes seems sensible. For hemodialysis patients, however, there is greater variability among clinicians in their preferred regimen. Current practice varies from 10–40 mg i.v. iron every dialysis session, to 100–200 mg once a week or fortnight. Both regimens are effective, and there are at present no comparative studies. It is impossible, therefore, to give firm recommendations for the optimal regimen at the present time. The likelihood, however, is that there is little difference between the various i.v. iron regimens; the important thing from a practical point of view is to recognize the potential development of functional iron deficiency and treat it aggressively with i.v. iron.

CAN AGGRESSIVE I.V. IRON SUPPLEMENTATION ENHANCE THE RESPONSE TO EPO AND REDUCE DOSAGE REQUIREMENTS?

Several published studies suggest that this may be the case, although most of them are small and uncontrolled, and include a significant number of iron-deficient patients (27–33). Macdougall et al. (27) randomized 37 patients starting EPO therapy to receive regular i.v. iron dextran (100 mg every 2 weeks), oral iron (ferrous sulfate 200 mg t.d.s.), or no iron. All were iron-replete (serum ferritin $>100\,\mu g/L$) at the start of the study. The i.v. iron-treated group had an enhanced hemoglobin response and better maintained ferritin levels, and required lower doses of EPO (27). Sunder-Plassmann and Horl (28) treated 52 hemodialysis patients with regular i.v. iron and obtained a rise in the hemoglobin from 9.4 ± 1.2 to 11.1 ± 1.1 g/dl and a 70% reduction in EPO dose (217 ± 179 to 62.6 ± 70.2 U/kg/week). Many of the patients in this study, however, were iron-deficient as judged by low serum ferritin levels. Similar findings were reported by Nyvad et al. (29), who, with regular i.v. iron hydroxysaccharate, maintained the hematocrit at a stable level (34.3% to 34.5%) but produced a

27% reduction in EPO dose from 6353 to 4586 U/week. Fishbane et al. (30) recently compared i.v. versus oral iron supplementation in 52 hemodialysis patients and observed a similar potentiation of hematocrit response ($32.5 \pm 0.6\%$ to $34.4 \pm 0.7\%$) and a reduction in EPO dosage requirements (7100 ± 571 to 4050 ± 634 U/treatment) in the group receiving i.v. iron. Studies by Al-Momen et al. (31), Silverberg et al. (32), and Taylor et al. (33) also provide data in support of aggressive i.v. iron supplementation.

CONCLUSIONS

Regular monitoring of iron status and consideration of the need for iron supplementation is mandatory in all patients treated with EPO. A baseline serum ferritin level is useful as a guide to the adequacy of iron stores, but once treatment with EPO has begun, this measurement is less helpful. Measurement of the percentage of hypochromic red cells is probably the best indicator of functional iron deficiency in patients receiving EPO, and values greater than 10% are strongly suggestive of this condition. The role of oral iron supplementation in patients treated with EPO is rather limited, since absorption from the gut is frequently inadequate to support the requirements of the marrow. As a result, many patients need i.v. iron supplementation, particularly in the correction phase of treatment. The choice of i.v. iron preparation is determined by several factors, including licensing availability in different countries, but iron hydroxysaccharate offers a good compromise in terms of readily available iron and a proven safety record. There is no universally recognized optimal regimen for giving i.v. iron at the present time, and comparative studies are required before firm recommendations can be given.

REFERENCES

1. Macdougall IC, Hutton RD, Cavill I, Coles GA, Williams JD. Poor response to treatment of renal anaemia with erythropoietin corrected by iron given intravenously. Br Med J 1989; 299:157–158.

2. Van Wyck DB, Stivelman JC, Ruiz J, Kirlin LF, Katz MA, Ogden DA. Iron status in patients receiving erythropoietin for dialysis associated anemia. Kidney Int 1989; 35:712–716.
3. Macdougall IC. Monitoring of iron status and iron supplementation in patients treated with erythropoietin. Curr Opinion Nephrol Hypertension 1994; 3:620–625.
4. Brozovich B, Cattell WR, Cottrall MF, Gwyther MM, McMillan JM, Malpas JS, Salsbury A, Trott NG. Iron metabolism in patients undergoing regular dialysis therapy. Br Med J 1971; 1:695–698.
5. Macdougall IC, Jones EA, Evans W, Cavill I, Coles GA, Williams JD. Measurement of occult gastrointestinal blood loss in haemodialysis patients on erythropoietin. Nephrol Dialysis Transplant 1993; 8:959.
6. Shepherd AMM, Stewart WK, Wormsley KG. Peptic ulceration in chronic renal failure. Lancet 1973; i:1357–1359.
7. Remuzzi G. Bleeding in renal failure. Lancet 1988; i:1205–1208.
8. Lindsay RM, Burton JA, Edward N, Dargie HJ, Prentice CRM, Kennedy AC. Dialyzer blood loss. Clin Nephrol 1973; 1:29–34.
9. Eschbach JW, Cook JD, Finch CA. Iron absorption in chronic renal disease. Clin Sci 1970; 38:191–196.
10. Milman N. Iron therapy in patients undergoing maintenance haemodialysis. Acta Med Scand 1976; 200:315–319.
11. Eschbach JW, Cook JD, Scribner BH. Iron balance in haemodialysis patients. Ann Intern Med 1977; 87:710–713.
12. Gokal R, Millard PR, Weatherall DJ, Callender STE, Ledingham JGG, Oliver DO. Iron metabolism in haemodialysis patients. Q J Med 1979; 48:369–391.
13. Cavill I. Diagnostic methods. Clinics in Haematology 1982; 11:259–273.
14. Eschbach JW, Egrie JC, Downing MR, Browne JK, Adamson JW. Correction of the anemia of end-stage renal disease with recombinant human erythropoietin. N Engl J Med 1987; 316:73–78.
15. Blumberg AB, Marti HRM, Graber CG. Serum ferritin and bone marrow iron in patients undergoing continuous ambulatory peritoneal dialysis. JAMA 1983; 250:3317–3319.
16. Bell JD, Kincaid WR, Morgan RG, Bunce H, Alperin JB, Sarles HE, Remmers AR. Serum ferritin assay and bone-marrow iron stores in patients on maintenance hemodialysis. Kidney Int 1980; 17:237–241.
17. Konijn AM, Hershko C. Ferritin synthesis in inflammation: pathogenesis of impaired iron release. Br J Haematol 1977; 37:7–16.
18. Birgegard G, Hallgren R, Killander A. Serum ferritin during infection: a longitudinal study. Scand J Haematol 1978; 21:333–340.

19. Macdougall IC, Hutton RD, Cavill I, Coles GA, Williams JD. Treating renal anaemia with recombinant human erythropoietin: practical guidelines and a clinical algorithm. Br Med J 1990; 300:655–659.
20. Rosenberg ME. Role of transferrin measurement in monitoring iron status during recombinant human erythropoietin therapy. Dialysis Transplant 1992; 21:81–90.
21. Bainton DF, Finch CA. The diagnosis of iron deficiency anemia. Am J Med 1964; 37:62–70.
22. Macdougall IC, Cavill I, Hulme B, Bain B, McGregor E, McKay P, Sanders E, Coles GA, Williams JD. Detection of functional iron deficiency during erythropoietin treatment: a new approach. Br Med J 1992; 304:225–226.
23. Brunati C, Piperno A, Guastoni C, Perrino ML, Civati G, Teatini U, Perego A, Fiorelli G, Minetti L. Erythrocyte ferritin in patients on chronic hemodialysis treatment. Nephron 1990; 54:219–223.
24. Garrett S, Worwood M. Zinc protoporphyrin and iron-deficient erythropoiesis. Acta Haematol 1994; 91:21–25.
25. Beguin Y, Loo M, R'Zik S, Sautois B, Lejeune F, Rorive G, Fillet G. Quantitative assessment of erythropoiesis in haemodialysis patients demonstrates gradual expansion of erythroblasts during constant treatment with recombinant human erythropoietin. Br J Haematol 1995; 89:17–23.
26. Geisser P, Baer M, Schaub E. Structure/histotoxicity relationship of parenteral iron preparations. Arzneim Forsch Drug Res 1992; 42:1439–1452.
27. Macdougall IC, Tucker B, Thompson J, Baker LRI, Raine AEG. A randomized controlled study of iron supplementation in patients treated with erythropoietin. Kidney Int 1996; 50:1694–1699.
28. Sunder-Plassmann G, Horl WH. Importance of iron supply for erythropoietin therapy. Nephrol Dialysis Transplant 1995; 10:2070–2076.
29. Nyvad O, Danielsen H, Madsen S. Intravenous iron-sucrose complex to reduce epoetin demand in dialysis patients. Lancet 1994; 344:1305–1306.
30. Fishbane S, Frei GL, Maesaka J. Reduction in recombinant human erythropoietin doses by the use of chronic intravenous iron supplementation. Am J Kidney Dis 1995; 26:41–46.
31. Al-Momen AM, Huraib SO, Mitwalli AH, Al-Wakeel J, Al-Yamani MJMS, Abu-Aisha H, Said R. Intravenous iron saccharate in hemodialysis patients receiving r-HuEPO. Saudi J Kidney Dis Transplant 1994; 5:168–172.

32. Silverberg DS, Blum M, Peer G, Kaplan E, Iaina A. Intravenous ferric saccharate as an iron supplement in dialysis patients. Nephron 1996; 72:413–417.
33. Taylor JE, Peat N, Porter C, Morgan AG. Regular intravenous iron therapy improves response to erythropoietin. Nephrol Dialysis Transplant 1996; 11:1428.

14

Continuous Administration of Intravenous Iron During Hemodialysis

C. Granolleras, A. Zein, R. Oulès, B. Branger, J. Fourcade, and S. Shaldon   University Hospital, Nîmes, France

INTRODUCTION

Intravenous iron was first administered to hemodialysis patients for treatment of anemia in 1965, when a policy of stopping blood transfusions was introduced. Even polytransfused, iron-overloaded patients responded with a rise in their hematocrit. The decision to pursue this apparently illogical procedure was due to a single observation. A polytransfused home-dialysis patient was being dialysed without water treatment in a Swiss village at an altitude of 2000 meters. Within 1 year after stopping blood transfusions, his hematocrit had risen to 40 vols%. A water-softener was introduced for water treatment, and his hematocrit fell to 28% and the iron deposits staining the dialysate tubes disappeared. On being given i.v. iron, his hematocrit rose to 48%. Following this serendipitous observation, one of us (S.S.) started to give i.v. iron to all hemodialysis patients and stopped all blood transfusions (1,2).

Many forms of i.v. iron are available throughout the world. However, because of side effects—occasionally fatal, and attributed to direct toxicity or to anaphylaxis or both—only certain preparations are available in certain countries (see Chapter 13). In France, only iron polymaltose (Fer Lucien®) is allowed, and only for patients on hemodialysis, and not even for continuous ambulatory peritoneal dialysis patients. Since 1977, we have given this iron mixed with heparin in saline as a continuous infusion via the syringe pump of the single-patient dialysate supply and monitoring unit.

Following the clinical introduction of erythropoietin (EPO) in 1986 (3), Eschbach and coworkers reported EPO resistance cured by i.v. iron in a single case report. Thereafter, the importance of giving i.v. iron to reduce EPO needs to reach target hematocrit levels became recognized. We demonstrated this benefit in a study showing a 30% reduction in EPO needs in a stable population on maintenance EPO (4). We describe below the technique that we recommend for the routine i.v. administration of iron in hemodialysis patients.

TECHNIQUE
Method of Administration

A vial of iron polymaltose containing 100 mg in a volume of 2 ml is drawn into a 2-ml syringe, and the appropriate dose of 10–100 mg is added to a 50-ml syringe containing 20 ml N saline and heparin (Heparin Choay® or Heparin Roch®) 2000–10000 units. The 20 ml is infused at a maximum rate of 7.5 ml/hr.

Pharmacological Compatibility

Physical

Microscopic particle counts at 5 minutes and 1, 5, 24, and 72 hours showed no increase over control (H. Woog, personal communication, 1996).

In Vivo Testing

Transferrin indices were measured at 14 days after a single dose of 100 mg iron and 5000 units of heparin were separately administered with two pumps and compared with the single-pumped mixture. No difference was observed in the transferrin saturation or ferritin levels.

Activated partial thromboplastin times (aPTT) were used as an index of heparin efficiency. Again, on separate administration there was no difference in the same patient when the heparin and iron were given together.

SUMMARY AND CONCLUSIONS

Continuous heparin and i.v. iron polymaltose can be given together without pharmacological incompatibility. Twenty years of experience in over 30,000 hemodialyses and more than 400 patients without a single adverse reaction suggest that this should be the method of choice. It allows the most controlled way of administration as well as being the most economical. It is available wherever one has a modern dialysis machine because the variable-speed syringe pump is a standard in all manufacturers' specifications. Thus, even without continuous heparinization, the technique can be utilized. Further work needs to be done to verify that other iron preparations are also pharmacologically compatible with heparin.

ACKNOWLEDGEMENT

We would like to thank Dr. Heinrich Woog, Head of the Galenical Development Division, Boehringer Mannheim GmbH, for his invaluable and prompt help in the evaluation of the physical compatibility study.

REFERENCES

1. Shaldon S. Chronic dialysis without transfusion [letter]. Lancet 1967; i: 783–784.
2. Crockett RE, Baillod RA, Lee BN, Moorhead JF, Stevenson CM, Varghese Z, Shaldon S. Maintenance of fifty patients on intermittent

haemodialysis without transfusion. Proceedings of the EDTA 1967; IV: 17–22.
3. Eschbach JW, Egrie JC, Downing MR, Browne JK, Adamson JW. Correction of the anemia of end-stage renal disease with recombinant human erythropoietin: results of a combined phase I and II clinical trial. N Engl J Med 1987; 316:73–78.
4. Granolleras C, Oulès R, Branger B, Fourcade J, Shaldon S. Iron supplementation of hemodialysis patients receiving recombinant human erythropoietin therapy. In: Bauer C, Koch KM, Scigalla P, Wieczorek L, eds. Erythropoietin: Molecular Physiology and Clinical Applications. New York: Marcel Dekker, 1993:211–216.

15

Erythropoietin and Kidney Transplantation

R. Vanholder and A. Van Loo   University Hospital, Ghent, Belgium

INTRODUCTION

The progression of renal failure is characterized by a progressive loss of the capacity of the kidneys to produce erythropoietin (EPO). This mechanism is one of the reasons that patients with end-stage renal failure develop invalidating anemia. Until a few years ago, except for blood transfusions, there existed no therapeutic modalities to correct this anemia, resulting in patient discomfort, effort intolerance, and an enhanced risk for ischemia-related cardiovascular complications. The development of recombinant human erythropoietin (rhEPO) made it possible to treat this condition in a safe and consistent way.

The first patient group that benefited from the availability of rhEPO were patients treated with chronic hemodialysis, followed by patients on continuous ambulatory peritoneal dialysis (CAPD). A patient group on renal replacement therapy that has been considered less for EPO treatment are kidney transplant recipients, especially since a normalization of red blood cell counts is observed in this population as soon as a few weeks after grafting. During follow-up, polycytemia is even observed in some patients.

In this chapter, we review various aspects of the influence of endogenous or recombinant EPO on the evolution of patients after renal transplantation. The following questions will be addressed:

1. Does the administration of rhEPO before renal transplantation affect the outcome of transplantation?
2. What is the endogenous EPO production in kidney-transplanted patients early after transplantation?
3. What is the role of endogenous EPO in posttransplantation polycytemia?
4. What is the effect of treatment with rhEPO in patients with chronic renal allograft rejection?
5. Is there a place for treatment with rhEPO during the first weeks after kidney transplantation?

DOES rhEPO ADMINISTRATION BEFORE RENAL TRANSPLANTATION AFFECT TRANSPLANTATION OUTCOME?

There are several theoretical reasons for assuming that the administration of rhEPO before kidney transplantation could affect outcome after transplantation (1–3). Some of these potential influencing factors would have a beneficial effect, while others would have a disadvantageous impact.

EPO has been associated with an increased risk for hypercoagulability (4) and improvement of immune response (5,6); these two factors might have a negative impact on the outcome after transplantation. It has been generally accepted that blood transfusions in the pretransplantation period improve tolerance of the grafted kidney, and hence outcome. As rhEPO obviates blood transfusion, this protective effect could be counteracted by EPO treatment. However, it has been stressed that pretransplantation transfusions have lost their primacy as a conditioning regimen with influence on posttransplantation outcome (7), perhaps because better preventive antirejection therapy became possible. On the other hand, rhEPO could eliminate the negative impact of repeated blood transfusions, such as the risk of transmission of infectious diseases (e.g., cytomegalic virus infection, hepatitis) and the deleterious toxic side effects of iron overload. Even more important, fewer blood transfusions could result in decreased development of lymphocytotoxic antibodies; it has been demonstrated that the presence of these antibodies is related to an increased risk of function loss of grafted kidneys within the year after transplantation (8).

Regarding HLA sensitization, it has been demonstrated that treatment with rhEPO results in a decrease in percentage of circulating panel reactive antibodies (PRA). In a study by Grimm et al. (9,10), an average decrease from $80 \pm 24\%$ before the start of rhEPO-treatment to 56 ± 41 after rhEPO was observed ($p < 0.05$). Similarly, Barany et al. (11) found a decrease from 60 to 35% ($p < 0.05$). Such decreases were not observed in all EPO-treated patients, however (12,13). The possibility should be considered that the most important benefit is observed in the mildly and moderately sensitized patients.

The first clinical observation to conform with the hypothesis that rhEPO before transplantation could have a negative impact on transplantation outcome was a case report by Zaoui et al. (14), who observed early kidney graft thrombosis in an EPO-treated patient. This hypothesis was apparently confirmed by a retrospective study by Schmidt et al. (15), who indicated that mean hematocrit at transplantation was lowest (27%) in the patients showing immediate graft function, intermediate (30%) in the patients showing delayed graft function, and highest (33%) in patients showing primary nonfunction. Careful analysis of these data, however, reveals that the most spectacular differences were observed in patients undergoing dialytic fluid removal immediately prior to transplantation. This impact of pretransplantation dialysis might be a confounding factor; its relative importance was not clearly considered in the abovementioned study. Consistent with the supposition that dialysis immediately prior to transplantation might have a negative impact on early graft function, it was demonstrated by the authors that patients undergoing hemodialysis, with a cuprophane membrane and/or with ultrafiltration of more than 500 ml, within 24 hours before transplantation were more prone to develop acute renal failure immediately after transplantation (16).

Other studies evaluating the impact of administration of rhEPO before transplantation on renal graft function could not corroborate the findings by Schmidt et al. and revealed no difference in early renal function up to 1 year after transplantation between EPO-treated and non-EPO-treated patients (17,18). Therefore, the impact of rhEPO on posttransplantation renal function is probably minimal to absent, although large-scale prospective studies are lacking.

WHAT IS THE ENDOGENOUS EPO PRODUCTION IN KIDNEY-TRANSPLANTED PATIENTS SOON AFTER TRANSPLANTATION?

Since a normally functioning kidney is implanted into a renal failure patient, it is conceivable that production of EPO will recover after kidney transplantation. The grafted kidney, however, does not always function perfectly in the weeks immediately following its implantation. The evolution is further obscured in the case of acute renal failure. Follow-up of serum EPO levels shows that there is a biphasic pattern. Shortly after transplantation, EPO levels are above normal; this can be attributed to EPO release from the kidney that has been damaged by its explanation and subsequent reimplantation. This is followed by normal to high-normal EPO levels during the next 3 to 4 weeks (19–21). These levels, although physiological for persons with a normal erythrocyte count, are too low for the hematocrits observed in the posttransplantation period, which may remain below 30% for several weeks (Figure 1) (21,22). Hence, a higher level of EPO would be needed to achieve normal erythropoiesis (23). EPO response might further be blunted in kidneys with delayed graft function (21), and in the case of iron deficiency (24). It is only after the first 3 to 4 weeks, in a second phase, that EPO levels gradually rise above normal values and hematocrit is normalized. If EPO levels are relatively low, improvement in hematocrit could be expected from the additional pharmacological administration of rhEPO in these patients. In chronic rejection patients, low endogenous EPO levels are associated with severe anemia (25).

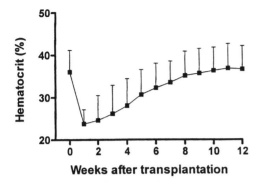

Figure 1   Evolution of the hematocrit during the first weeks after kidney transplantation (no EPO treatment). There is a progressive decrease from transplantation on, with a nadir after the first week (Hct = 23.8 ± 3.4%) (n = 16). Then a gradual recovery occurs. However, Hct >36% is reached only at the tenth week.

WHAT IS THE ROLE OF ENDOGENOUS EPO IN POSTTRANSPLANTATION POLYCYTEMIA?

Some transplanted patients suffer from erythrocytosis (26), and this condition is sometimes but not always associated with increased circulating EPO levels (27).

Whereas posttransplantation erythrocytosis was originally treated with repeated phlebotomy, it appeared later that medical treatment with angiotensin-converting enzyme (ACE) inhibitors also had a beneficial effect (27–29). It has been thought that this effect of ACE inhibitors could be related to the known property of angiotensin to stimulate EPO production, so that, conceivably, ACE inhibitors would depress EPO release. Later studies demonstrated, however, that during treatment with ACE inhibitors, hematocrit decreased in spite of EPO levels that remained elevated, suggesting EPO resistance (29). Consistent with this observation, we found that administration of ACE inhibitors was also related to depressed hematocrits in EPO-treated hemodialysis patients (30), in whom EPO resistance is much more conceivable as a mechanism than decreased production.

It has been claimed that transplanted patients who received EPO prior to transplantation would develop less erythrocytosis (31).

WHAT IS THE EFFECT OF rhEPO TREATMENT IN PATIENTS WITH CHRONIC RENAL ALLOGRAFT REJECTION?

Patients with chronic graft rejection progressively develop renal failure. Administration of rhEPO is as useful here as in any other variety of chronic renal failure (32,33). Treatment has no influence on the evolution of renal function.

IS THERE A PLACE FOR rhEPO TREATMENT DURING THE FIRST WEEKS AFTER KIDNEY TRANSPLANTATION?

Very few data are available regarding the efficacy of rhEPO during the first weeks after kidney transplantation. In one report (3), a recently transplanted patient with acute renal failure was successfully treated with EPO. The question arises as to whether rhEPO administered in doses currently used in renal failure patients will be able to cause a rise in serum EPO and hence in erythrocyte reactivity in the immediate posttransplantation period. Pharmacokinetic studies on the fate of rhEPO injected subcutaneously in chronic renal failure patients demonstrate that levels in the range of 100 U/ml are easily reached (34,35), which is markedly higher than the range of 25–30 U/ml resulting from endogenous production after transplantation (1). Therefore, on pharmacokinetic grounds, it can be expected that subcutaneous EPO after transplantation will cause sufficiently important changes in circulating EPO levels to influence erythropoiesis.

We recently completed a randomized, open, prospective trial comparing transplanted patients treated with rhEPO with those not so treated (36). EPO administration was started when posttransplantation hematocrit fell below 30%. The study revealed a significantly higher and faster rise in hematocrit in the EPO-treated patients

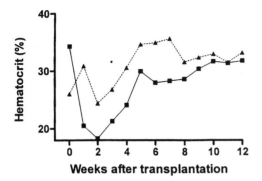

Figure 2 Evolution of the hematocrit in two representative patients, one treated with EPO after transplantation (solid line) and the other not (broken line).

(Figure 2) in spite of a number of factors that could affect hematocrit negatively in the EPO-treated group, such as: 1) a lower starting hematocrit value, 2) a higher incidence of major complications, and 3) fewer blood transfusions. Higher quantities of EPO were to be administered, compared to before transplantation. The response to EPO was blunted in patients developing major complications after their transplantation (surgical reintervention, CMV infection, sepsis).

   After completion of the study and analysis of the data, it became clear that modifications in the approach might have a further beneficial effect on the outcome: 1) rhEPO was started only when hematocrit fell below 30%; since a hematocrit fall is almost inevitable in these patients, it seems more logical to start or continue EPO treatment immediately after transplantation; 2) the dose was increased only gradually as a function of the hematocrit, and a more aggressive approach in the adaptation of the dose might have a positive influence on hematocrit; and 3) iron was administered only orally, and a serum ferritin of only 50 ng/ml was pursued; more vigorous, eventually intravenous, administration of iron, immediately after surgery, and the extension of the threshold ferritin to 200 ng/ml may also cause an additional benefit. A new prospective protocol is being developed in an attempt to avoid these pitfalls.

Another potential benefit of EPO after transplantation might be related to the prevention or reduction of early graft dysfunction. It has recently been demonstrated by Vaziri et al. (37) that EPO has a beneficial effect on renal function in cisplatin-induced acute renal failure in the rat. The authors could find no difference in renal function parameters between EPO-treated and non-EPO-treated renal transplant patients. However, the number of patients enrolled and the incidence of early graft dysfunction were too low to allow any definite conclusion.

It might be argued that the continued administration of EPO after transplantation may add an extra financial burden, but it should be realized that prolonged anemia after transplantation may carry its own morbidity and mortality. Anemia may be a source of more concern at present, since the enrollment of patients on the transplantation waiting list becomes less and less restrictive; the prognosis of these patients is jeopardized by a higher risk of ischemic complications. Moreover, blood transfusions are administered only reluctantly, in view of their capacity to trigger the formation of lymphocytotoxic antibodies and the transmission of viral infections.

CONCLUSIONS

EPO treatment before renal transplantation probably has no negative effect on the outcome. On the contrary, it reduces the concentration of circulating lymphocytotoxic antibodies, and may hence have a beneficial effect on long-term outcome, especially in intermediately sensitized patients.

Although circulating EPO levels normalize shortly after transplantation, it is insufficient to correct erythrocyte counts, suggesting EPO resistance.

EPO may play a role in posttransplantation erythrocytosis, although this remains a matter of debate. This condition can be easily treated with ACE inhibitors, although the mechanism remains a matter of debate.

rhEPO is helpful to correct anemia in chronic rejection. Recent data collected by the authors suggest that EPO may also be of benefit when administered immediately after transplantation. In addition, EPO could counteract the development or maintenance of acute renal graft failure.

REFERENCES

1. Ward HJ. Implications of recombinant erythropoietin therapy for renal transplantation. Am J Nephrol 1990; 10(suppl 2):44–52.
2. Moore R. Towards long-term graft survival in renal transplantation: the role of erythropoietin. Nephrol Dialysis Transplant 1995; 10(suppl 1):20–22.
3. Ettenger RB, Marik J, Grimm P. The impact of recombinant human erythropoietin on renal transplantation. Am J Kidney Dis 1991; 18: 57–61.
4. Clyne N, Lins LE, Egberg N. Long-term effects of erythropoietin treatment on the coagulation system during standardized hemodialysis. Clin Nephrol 1995; 43:260–267.
5. Veys N, Vanholder R, Ringoir S. Correction of deficient phagocytosis during erythropoietin (EPO) treatment in maintenance haemodialysis patients. Am J Kidney Dis 1992; 19:358–363.
6. Vanholder R, Ringoir S. Infectious morbidity and defects of phagocytic function in end-stage renal disease: a review. J Am Soc Nephrol 1993; 3:1541–1554.
7. Opelz G. HLA antigen sensitization: a problem in graft survival. Transplant Proc 1989; 21:39–41.
8. Opelz G, Graver B, Mickey MR, Terasaki PI. Lymphocytotoxic antibody responses to transfusions in potential kidney transplant recipients. Transplantation 1981; 32:177–183.
9. Grimm PC, Sekiya NM, Robertson LS, Robinson BJ, Ettenger RB. Recombinant human erythropoietin decreases anti-HLA sensitization and may improve renal allograft outcome: involvement of anti-idiotypic antibody. Transplant Proc 1991; 23:407–408.
10. Grimm PC, Sinai-Triemen L, Sekiya NM, Robertson LS, Robinson BJ, Fine RN, Ettenger RB. Effects of recombinant human erythropoietin on HLA sensitization and cell mediated immunity. Kidney Int 1990; 38:12–18.
11. Barany P, Fehrman I, Godoy C. Long-term effects on lymphocytotoxic antibodies and immune reactivity in hemodialysis patients treated with recombinant human erythropoietin. Clin Nephrol 1992; 37:90–96.

12. Phelan DL, Hibbett S, Wetter L, Hanto DW, Mohanakumar T. Recombinant erythropoietin: does it really effect sensitization? Transplant Proc 1991; 23:409–410.
13. Koskimies S, Lautenschlager I, Grönhagen-Riska C, Häyry P. Erythropoietin therapy and the antibody levels of highly sensitized patients awaiting kidney transplantation. Transplantation 1990; 50:707–709.
14. Zaoui P, Bayle F, Maurizi J, Foret M, DalSoglio S, Vialtel P. Early thrombosis in kidney grafted into patients treated with erythropoietin [letter]. Lancet 1988; ii:956.
15. Schmidt R, Kupin W, Dumler F, Venkat KK, Mozes M. Influence of the pretransplant hematocrit level on early graft function in primary cadaveric renal transplantation. Transplantation 1993; 55:1034–1040.
16. Vanholder R, Bernaert P, Van Loo A, Lameire N, Ringoir S. Pre-transplant (TP) hemodialysis (HD) with cuprophane (CUP) and/or ultrafiltration (UF) decreases early graft function [abstr]. J Am Soc Nephrol 1994; 5:482.
17. Paganini EP, Braun WE, Latham D, Abdulhadi MH. Renal transplantation: results in hemodialysis patients previously treated with recombinant human erythropoietin. ASAIO Trans 1989; 35:535–538.
18. Linde T, Wahlberg J, Wikström B, Danielson BG. Outcome of renal transplantation in patients treated with erythropoietin. Clin Nephrol 1992; 37:260–263.
19. Sun CH, Ward HJ, Paul WL, Koyle MA, Yanagawa N, Lee DBN. Serum erythropoietin levels after renal transplantation. N Engl J Med 1989; 321:151–157.
20. Soh S, Kumano K, Utsunomiya T, Mashimo S, Endo T. Serum erythropoietin levels after renal transplantation. Transplant Proc 1994; 26: 2154–2156.
21. Moulin B, Ollier J, George F, Purgus R, Roux F, Sampol J, Olmer M. Serum erythropoietin and reticulocyte maturity index after renal transplantation: a prospective longitudinal study. Nephron 1995; 69:259–266.
22. Goch J, Birgegard G, Wikström B, Tufveson G, Danielson BG. Serum erythropoietin levels in the immediate kidney-posttransplant period. Nephron 1992; 60:30–34.
23. Morel P, Hadj-Aïssa A, Pouteil-Noble C, Touraine JL, Pozet N. Long-term evolution of erythropoietin after successful renal transplantation [letter]. Nephron 1993; 64:491–492.
24. Moore LW, Smith SO, Winsett RP, Acchiardo SR, Gaber AO. Factors affecting erythropoietin production and correction of anemia in kidney transplant recipients. Clin Transplant 1994; 8:358–364.

25. Heidenreich S, Tepel M, Fahrenkamp A, Rahn KH. Prognostic value of serum erythropoietin levels in late acute rejection of renal transplants. Am J Kidney Dis 1995; 25:775–780.

26. Sumrani NB, Daskalakis P, Miles AM, Sarkar S, Markell MS, Hong JH, Friedman EA, Sommer BG. Erythrocytosis after renal transplantation: a prospective analysis. ASAIO J 1993; 39:51–55.

27. Danovitch GM, Jamgotchian NJ, Eggena PH, Paul W, Barrett JD, Wilkinson A, Lee DBN. Angiotensin-converting enzyme inhibition in the treatment of renal transplant erythrocytosis. Transplantation 1995; 60: 132–137.

28. Torregrosa JV, Campistol JM, Montesinos M, Rogada AG, Oppenheimer F, Andreu J. Efficacy of captopril on posttransplant erythrocytosis. Transplantation 1994; 58:311–314.

29. Perazella M, MacPhedran P, Kliger A, Lorber M, Levy E, Bia MJ. Enalapril treatment of posttransplant erythrocytosis: efficacy independent of circulating erythropoietin levels. Am J Kidney Dis 1995; 26: 495–500.

30. Dhondt AW, Vanholder RC, Ringoir SMG. Angiotensin-converting enzyme inhibitors and higher erythropoietin requirement in chronic hemodialysis patients. Nephrol Dialysis Transplant 1995; 10:2107–2109.

31. Kessler M, Legrand E, Mertes M, Renoult E, Hestin D. Treatment of chronic renal failure anemia by recombinant erythropoietin and polycythemia following kidney transplantation [letter]. Nephron 1992; 62: 370–371.

32. Muirhead N, Cattran DC, Zaltzman J, Jindal K, First MR, Boucher A, Keown PA, Munch LC, Wong C. Safety and efficacy of recombinant human erythropoietin in correcting the anemia of patients with chronic renal allograft dysfunction. J Am Soc Nephrol 1994; 5:1216–1222.

33. Sanaka T, Takahashi K, Teraoka S, Toma H, Agishi T, Sugino N, Ota K. Usefulness of protein-restricted diet and recombinant human erythropoietin in patients with chronic rejection of a transplanted kidney. Transplant Proc 1992; 4:1571–1572.

34. Ateshkadi A, Johnson CA, Oxton LL, Hammond TG, Bohenek WS, Zimmerman SW. Pharmacokinetics of intraperitoneal, intravenous, and subcutaneous recombinant human erythropoietin in patients on continuous ambulatory peritoneal dialysis. Am J Kidney Dis 1993; 21: 635–642.

35. Brockmöller J, Köchling J, Weber W, Looby M, Roots J, Neumayer HH. The pharmacokinetics of recombinant human erythropoietin in haemodialysis patients. Br J Clin Pharmacol 1992; 34:499–508.

36. Van Loo A, Vanholder R, Bernaert P, De Roose J, Lameire N. Recombinant human erythropoietin corrects anaemia during the first weeks after renal transplantation: a randomized prospective study. Nephrol Dialysis Transplant 1996; 11:1815–1821.
37. Vaziri ND, Zhou XJ, Liao SY. Erythropoietin enhances recovery from cisplatin-induced acute renal failure. Am J Physiol 1994; 35: F360–F366.

16

Effects of rhEPO on Regulation of Pulsatile Gonadotropin Secretion

Franz Schaefer and Birgit van Kaick   Children's Hospital and University of Heidelberg, Heidelberg, Germany

Günter Stein   Friedrich-Schiller University of Jena, Jena, Germany

Eberhard Ritz   Ruperto Carola University, Heidelberg, Germany

SUMMARY

Treatment with recombinant human erythropoietin (rhEPO) improves reproductive functions in patients with end-stage renal failure. An increase in sex-steroid concentrations has been reported more often than not, but no consistent effect on baseline or stimulated gonadotropin concentrations has been demonstrated. To determine whether rhEPO might induce any changes in the temporal pattern and biopotency of pulsatile luteinizing hormone (LH) secretion, we evaluated plasma hormone concentration profiles in seven hemodialyzed men before and after partial correction of anemia. During rhEPO treatment, distinct changes occurred in secretion and elimination rates as well as relative biopotency of LH, despite no change in *mean* plasma hormone concentrations. Mean half-life of plasma LH disappearance decreased by 38%, while the mass of LH secreted per burst and the total LH secretion rate doubled during partial correction of anemia. The resulting plasma concentration profile exhibited was more distinctly pulsatile, as expressed by an increase in the fractional amplitude of bio-LH concentration pulses. The proportion of bioactive LH isoforms increased, as suggested by a rising ratio of bioactive to immunoreactive LH. In conclusion, rhEPO treatment causes 1) an increased activity of the hypothalamopituitary unit under rhEPO treatment, 2) a decrease in the plasma half-life of bio-LH, and 3) greater LH signal strength delivered to the target tissue as a result of an increased mass per burst and incremental amplitude of the plasma concentration pattern.

DISORDERS OF GONADOTROPIN SECRETION IN CHRONIC RENAL FAILURE

Altered sexual function is a frequent complication of chronic renal failure (CRF). In male patients, reduced libido, potentia, and fertility have been reported (1). Plasma gonadotropins are high-normal or elevated, and plasma androgens decreased or low-normal (2). The elevation of plasma LH levels is due in significant part to the reduced metabolic clearance rate and prolonged plasma half-life of the hormone (3,4). Indeed, mathematical modeling of the pulsatile plasma concentration patterns has shown that LH secretion rates are reduced despite elevated mean circulating concentrations (5,6). Experimental in vitro (7) and in vivo (8) studies suggest diminished release of gonadotropin-releasing hormone (GnRH) from the hypothalamus in uremia. The increase in plasma LH levels in response to an exogenous bolus of GnRH is blunted but prolonged (9–11); however, the actual secretory reserve capacity of the pituitary, as calculated by allowing for prolonged LH half-life, is normal (5). These observations suggest a primary alteration of the hypothalamopituitary unit and/or its feedback regulation in uremia. Moreover, the biological activity of circulating LH, i.e., the potency of a given mass of immunoreactive hormone to induce testosterone release from

Leydig cells, is impaired in adolescent and adult patients on dialysis (12–14). Since bioactive LH isoforms may enter the circulation preferentially during GnRH-stimulated secretory episodes (15), reduced LH bioactivity in uremia may be interpreted as being further evidence for insufficient release of GnRH from the hypothalamic pulse generator.

EFFECTS OF rhEPO ON REPRODUCTIVE FUNCTION

The correction of anemia in renal failure by rhEPO treatment improves several functions that are coordinated at the hypothalamic level, such as appetite (16–18) and sexual activity (16,19,20). The endocrine mechanism of the improvement of sexual functions is unclear. Most studies were not able to demonstrate consistent changes in plasma LH concentrations, either collected as random samples under basal conditions or after stimulation with supramaximal exogenous GnRH boli, under rhEPO treatment (18,19,21,22). However, in men with hypotestosteronemia, partial normalization of plasma testosterone levels during rhEPO treatment has been reported (18,23, 24). These findings suggest an improved sensitivity of Leydig cells to simulation by LH.

IMPORTANCE AND ASSESSMENT OF EPISODIC GONADOTROPIN SECRETION

The gonadotropins are secreted in an episodic (pulsatile) fashion, with an average frequency in adult men of one plasma concentration pulse per 90 minutes. The pulsatile release of LH mirrors intermittent GnRH bursts arriving in the pituitary after synchronous release from highly specialized neurons in the hypothalamus, the so-called GnRH pulse generator. The pulsatile mode of GnRH release is vital to prevent down-regulation of GnRH receptors in the pituitary (25). In analogy, the pulsatile LH signal may be of relevance to the end-organ tissue, the Leydig cells, as a fast, efficient, and economic way of interglandular communication.

We and others (5,6) have reported alterations of spontaneous pulsatile LH secretion in uremic individuals. With respect to the possible endocrine mechanisms underlying the clinical improvement of reproductive functions, we hypothesized that rhEPO treatment might quantitatively and/or qualitatively normalize the abnormalities of spontaneous pulsatile gonadotropin secretion in uremia. Such changes would not be detected by routine random blood sampling, but require an assessment of the plasma concentration patterns of LH by frequent blood sampling. Moreover, we assessed possible changes in the relative biopotency of LH (bio-LH) by using an in vitro Leydig cell bioassay (26) in combination with standard radioimmunological measurement. Finally, the hormone concentration vs. time series were analyzed by a sophisticated multiparameter algorithm (deconvolution analysis), which permitted us to quantitate and differentiate the rates of hormone secretion into and elimination from the distribution space (27). More specifically, our deconvolution approach assumed that the plasma concentrations of bio-LH at any given instant result from the simultaneous operation of four distinct secretory and clearance terms: 1) the number, 2) the amplitudes, and 3) the durations of all prior (LH) secretory impulses, acted upon by 4) endogenous clearance kinetics.

Plasma hormone concentration profiles were obtained in seven adult hemodialyzed men both before and after partial correction of renal anemia by rhEPO. After 8 hours of blood sampling at 10-minute intervals, a supramaximal intravenous bolus of GnRH was administered, and plasma LH measurements continued for another 4 hours. The detailed results of this study have been published elsewhere (28).

CHANGES IN GONADOTROPIN KINETICS

The plasma disappearance half-life of bio-LH decreased by 40%, from 106 ± 10 minutes to 67 ± 7.2 minutes. The combined analysis of all studies (pre- and posttreatment) showed a significant inverse association between bio-LH half-life and hematocrit ($r = -0.83$; $p < 0.02$) (Figure 1). This finding may be explained by the pharmaco-

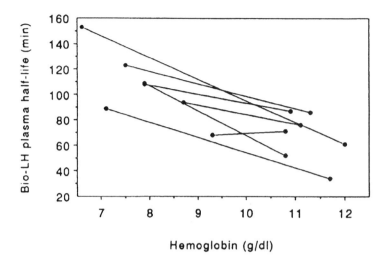

Figure 1 Relationship between changes in hematocrit levels and plasma half-life of bio-LH during partial correction of renal anemia by rhEPO treatment. (From Ref. 28.)

kinetic definition of the relationship between hormone distribution and elimination, which is given by the equation half-life equals ln 2 times the volume of distribution, divided by the metabolic clearance rate. While a reduction in metabolic clearance rate for LH is well established in uremic animals (3) and humans (4), less attention has been paid to alterations in the volume of distribution of the hormone. The apparent distribution space of LH is determined mainly by the size of the plasma volume. To maintain a constant intravascular volume, subjects with longstanding anemia adapt to the reduced total red cell mass by an expansion of their plasma volume. Thus, the apparent volume of LH distribution in an individual with anemia of renal origin should be increased. The correction of anemia by rhEPO treatment results in an expansion of the total red cell mass, which is compensated for by simultaneous shrinking of the extracellular fluid space (29), presumably mainly of the plasma volume. As a consequence, the apparent volume of LH distribution is likely to decline

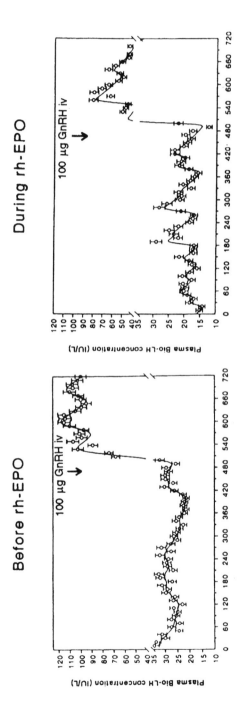

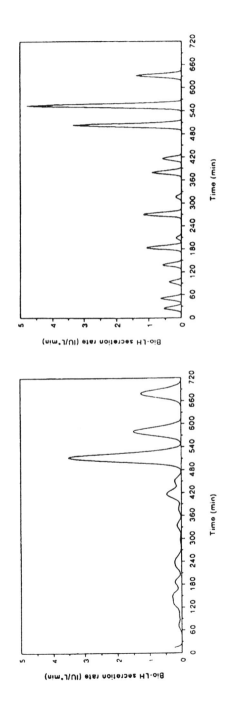

Figure 2 Plasma biologically active LH concentration vs. time profiles before and during rhEPO treatment, analyzed by multiparameter deconvolution techniques. Samples were obtained at 10-minute intervals between 08.00 and 20.00 hours. After 8 hours, an i.v. bolus of GnRH (100 μg) was administered. Upper panels depict measured bioactive LH values (mean ± SD of duplicate measurements) and fitted curves; lower panels give deconvolution-estimated secretion rates. LH bioactivity was determined in the mouse Leydig cell bioassay. (From Ref. 28.)

during rhEPO treatment. On the basis of this relationship, the observed decrease in plasma LH half-life and the close inverse association between the changes in plasma half-life and hematocrit can be explained largely by a reduction of the apparent distribution space in response to rhEPO treatment.

QUANTITATIVE CHANGES IN LH SECRETION

Figure 2 shows the application of deconvolution analysis to the concentration vs. time series of bio-LH in a representative patient. Although the mean plasma concentrations of bio-LH did not change, the average rate of spontaneous bio-LH secretion approximately doubled under rhEPO treatment. This increase was attributable to a twofold increase of the hormone mass secreted within each burst of bio-LH, whereas the frequency of secretory episodes remained unchanged. The augmentation of bio-LH burst mass was related to a tendency for an increased burst amplitude rather than a change in burst duration. The average fractional amplitude of the plasma concentration pulses increased in all but one patient, from a mean of 112 to 121%. In the 4 hours after administration of a supramaximal bolus of GnRH, two to five secretory episodes of bio-LH of high amplitude were observed. The absolute GnRH-stimulated bio-LH production rate was similar before and after rhEPO administration. The relative increase in bio-LH secretion rate after GnRH stimulation was reduced, however, from 380 to 190% of baseline secretion rate.

The observed doubling of LH secretion rate may be interpreted as being a physiological response to the shortening of plasma half-life induced by the partial correction of anemia. In a feedback-controlled homeostatic system, the decrease in plasma half-life should stimulate LH secretion rates in order to keep average plasma LH concentrations constant. In principle, the rise of LH secretion rate may be explained either by enhanced pituitary responsiveness to stimulation by GnRH or by an increased activity of the GnRH pulse generator. The stimulated LH release after a supramaximal exogenous bolus of GnRH did not change in response to rhEPO treatment. This finding suggests no change in pituitary responsiveness, at least to supramaximal doses of GnRH.

Animal experiments have recently provided in vitro and in vivo evidence of reduced hypothalamic GnRH secretion as the likely primary alteration underlying the diminished LH release in uremia (7, 8). Therefore, although we cannot exclude a subtle improvement of the gonadotroph responsiveness to physiological endogenous pulses of GnRH, the increase in LH production is more likely to reflect a trend toward normalization of hypothalamic GnRH release. Electrophysiological and cognitive performance studies have demonstrated an improvement of global central nervous function under rhEPO treatment (30,31). Hypothalamic "recovery" may also occur, with an impact not only on the hypothalamo-pituitary-gonadotropic axis, but also on appetite, libido, and memory. At present, it is not known whether the central nervous effects of rhEPO are due to improved tissue oxygenation, tropic actions, or rheological changes, or more generally to increased physical activity, reversal of malnutrition, and changes in lifestyle.

QUALITATIVE CHANGES IN LH SECRETION

Whereas the mean plasma bio-LH concentrations did not change during treatment, the concentrations of immunoreactive LH decreased significantly. Consequently, the ratios of bioactive to immunoreactive plasma LH concentrations increased. This apparent shift toward a greater proportion of more bioactive LH isoforms in the circulation may be a consequence of the putative increase in pulsatile GnRH secretion, since the release of bioactive LH molecules is apparently coupled to the periods of maximal endogenous GnRH secretion (15). Alternatively, rhEPO decreased the half-life of immunoreactive LH more than that of bioactive hormone.

CHANGES IN TESTICULAR RESPONSIVENESS
TO LH SIGNAL

Total plasma testosterone concentrations tended to increase during rhEPO treatment. Sex-hormone binding globulin (SHBG) levels decreased, resulting in a marked increase of the testosterone-SHBG ratio. Assuming no change in the dissociation constants, these changes should result in a commensurate increase in free plasma testosterone concentrations. Thus, the observed quantitative and qualitative changes in LH secretion during rhEPO treatment—i.e., the restoration of a pulsatile pattern of plasma LH fluctuations and the relative shift toward a higher proportion of bioactive LH isoforms available at the receptor site—may indeed have contributed to an improved target tissue response. Further possible mechanisms to explain the rise in free plasma testosterone include an improved secretory capacity of the Leydig cells as a result of better tissue oxygenation and/or nutritional status.

REFERENCES

1. Lim V. Reproductive function in patients with renal insufficiency. Am J Kidney Dis 1987; 9:363–367.
2. Handelsman DJ. Hypothalamic-pituitary gonadal dysfunction in renal failure, dialysis and renal transplantation. Endocr Rev 1985; 6:151–182.
3. Gay VL. Decreased metabolism and increased serum concentrations of LH and FSH following nephrectomy of the rat: absence of short-loop regulatory mechanism. Endocrinology 1974; 95:1582–1588.
4. Holdsworth S, Atkins R, de Kretser D. The pituitary-testicular axis in men with chronic renal failure. N Engl J Med 1977; 296:1245–1249.
5. Veldhuis JD, Wilkowski MJ, Zwart AD, et al. Evidence for attenuation of hypothalamic gonadotropin-releasing hormone (GnRH) impulse strength with preservation of GnRH pulse frequency in men with chronic renal failure. J Clin Endocrinol Metab 1993; 76:648–654.
6. Schaefer F, Veldhuis JD, Robertson WR, Dunger D, Schaerer K. The Cooperative Study Group on Pubertal Development in Chronic Renal Failure. Immunoreactive and bioactive luteinizing hormone in pubertal patients with chronic renal failure. Kidney Int 1994; 45:1465–1476.
7. Wibullaksanakul S, Handelsman DJ. Regulation of hypothalamic gonadotropin-releasing hormone secretion in experimental uremia: in vitro studies. Neuroendocrinology 1991; 54:353–358.
8. Schaefer F, Daschner M, Veldhuis JD, Oh J, Qadri F, Schaerer K. In vivo alterations in the gonadotropic releasing hormone (GnRH) pulse

generator, and the secretion and clearance of luteinizing hormone in the castrate uremic rat. Neuroendocrinology 1994; 59:285–296.
9. Mies R, von Bayer H, Figge H, Finke K, Winkelmann W. Investigations on pituitary and Leydig cell function in chronic hemodialysis and after renal transplantation. Klin Wschr 1975; 53:611–615.
10. Gomez F, de la Cueva R, Wauters J-P, Lemarchand-Béraud T. Endocrine abnormalities in patients undergoing long-term hemodialysis. Am J Med 1980; 68:522–530.
11. Kawamura J, Daijyo K, Hosokawa S, Sawanishi K, Yoshida O, Oseko F. Hypothalamo-pituitary-testicular axis in men undergoing chronic intermittent hemodialysis. Int J Artif Organs 1978; 1:224–230.
12. Talbot JA, Rodger RSC, Robertson WR. Pulsatile bioactive luteinising hormone secretion in men with chronic renal failure and following renal transplantation. Nephron 1990; 56:66–72.
13. Schaefer F, Seidel C, Mitchell R, Schärer K, Robertson WR: The Cooperative Study Group on Pubertal Development In Chronic Renal Failure. Pulsatile immunoreactive and bioactive luteinizing hormone secretion in pubertal patients with chronic renal failure. Pediatr Nephrol 1991; 5:566–571.
14. Giusti M, Perfumo F, Verrina E, Cavallero D, Piaggio G, Gusmano R, Giordano G. Biological activity of luteinizing hormone in uremic children: spontaneous nocturnal secretion and changes after administration of exogenous pulsatile luteinizing hormone releasing hormone. Pediatr Nephrol 1991; 5:559–565.
15. Veldhuis JD, Johnson ML, Dufau ML. Preferential release of bioactive luteinizing hormone in response to endogenous and low dose exogenous gonadotropin-releasing hormone pulses in man. J Clin Endocrinol Metab 1987; 64:1275–1282.
16. Bommer J, Alexiou C, Müller-Bühl U, Eifert J, Ritz E. Recombinant human erythropoietin therapy in hemodialysis patients—dose determination and clinical experience. Nephrol Dialysis Transplant 1987; 2:238–242.
17. Eschbach JW, Kelly MR, Haley NR, Abels RI, Adamson JW. Treatment of the anemia of progressive renal failure with recombinant human erythropoietin. N Engl J Med 1989; 321:158–163.
18. Ramirez G, Bittle PA, Sanders H, Bercu BB. Hypothalamo-hypophyseal thyroid and gonadal function before and after erythropoietin therapy in dialysis patients. J Clin Endocrinol Metab 1992; 75:517–524.
19. Bommer J, Kugel M, Schwöbel B, Ritz E, Barth HP. Improved sexual function during recombinant human erythropoietin therapy. Nephrol Dialysis Transplant 1990; 5:204–207.

20. Sobh MA, Abd el Hamid IA, Gehad Atta M, Refaie AF. Effect of erythropoietin on sexual potency in chronic hemodialysis patients. Scand J Urol Nephrol 1992; 26:181–185.
21. Kokot F, Wiecek A, Grzeszczak W, Klepacka J, Klin M, Lao M. Influence of erythropoietin treatment on endocrine abnormalities in hemodialysis patients. Contrib Nephrol 1989; 76:257–272.
22. Watschinger B, Watschinger U, Templ H, Spona J, Graf H, Luger A. Effect of recombinant human erythropoietin on anterior pituitary function in patients on chronic hemodialysis. Horm Res 1991; 36:22–26.
23. Kokot F, Wiecek A, Greszczak W, Klepacka J, Klin M, Lao M. Influence of erythropoietin treatment on endocrine abnormalities in hemodialyzed patients. Contrib Nephrol 1989; 76:257–272.
24. Haley NR, Matsumoto AM, Eschbach JW, Adamson JM. Low testosterone levels increase in male hemodialysis patients treated with recombinant human erythropoietin. Kidney Int 1989; 35:193–196.
25. Crowley W, Filicori M, Spratt D, Santoro N. The physiology of gonadotropin-releasing hormone (GnRH) secretion in men and women. Recent Prog Horm Res 1985; 41:473–531.
26. Robertson WR, Bidey SP. The in vitro bioassay of peptide hormones. In: Hutton JC, Siddle K, eds. Peptide Hormone Secretion: A Practical Approach. Oxford: IRL Press, 1990:121–157.
27. Veldhuis JD, Carlson ML, Johnson ML. The pituitary gland secretes in bursts: appraising the nature of glandular secretory impulses by simultaneous multiple-parameter deconvolution of plasma hormone concentrations. Proc Natl Acad Sci USA 1987; 84:7686–7690.
28. Schaefer F, van Kaick B, Veldhuis JD, Stein G, Schaerer K, Robertson WR, Ritz E. Changes in the kinetics and biopotency of luteinizing hormone in hemodialyzed men during treatment with recombinant human erythropoietin. J Am Soc Nephrol 1994; 5:1208–1215.
29. Abraham PA, Opsahl J, Keshaviah PK, Collins AJ, Whalen JJ, Asinger RW, McLain LA, Hanson G, Davis MG, Halstenson CE. Body fluid spaces and blood pressure in hemodialysis patients during amelioration of anemia with erythropoietin. Am J Kid Dis 1990; 16:428–446.
30. Marsh JT, Brown WS, Wolcott D, Carr CR, Harper R, Schweitzer SV, Nissenson AR. rHuEPO treatment improves brain and cognitive function of anemic dialysis patients. Kidney Int 1991; 39:155–163.
31. Di Paolo B, Di Liberato L, Fiederling B, Catucci G, Bucciarelli S, Paolantonio L, Albertazzi A. Effects of uremia and dialysis on brain electrophysiology after recombinant erythropoietin (r-HuEPO). ASAIO J 1992; 38:M477–M480.

17

Anemia Correction and Cardiac Function
Coronary Artery Disease and Left-Ventricular Hypertrophy

V. Wizemann   Georg-Haas-Dialysezentrum, Giessen, Germany

INTRODUCTION

Cardiovascular complications are the most frequent cause of death in dialysis patients, and the risk of cardiac death in this patient group is increased about 20-fold as compared to the general population (1). The two main cardiac diseases prevalent in dialysis patients are coronary artery disease (CAD) and left ventricular hypertrophy (LVH), both of which can result in periods of myocardial ischemia. As shown in Figure 1, ischemia periods on electrocardiogram (ECG) are more frequent in dialysis patients with either LVH or CAD than in a group of end-stage renal disease (ESRD) patients who have normal hearts when studied by echocardiography and coronary angiography. In clinical praxis, both cardiac diseases are often coexisting and overt angina pectoris can be observed in about 20% of dialysis patients during dialysis (2).

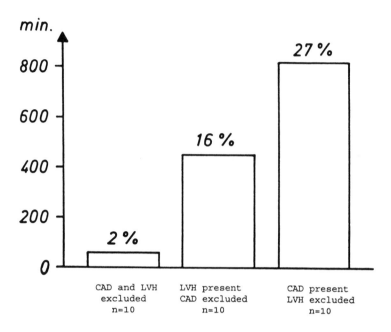

Figure 1   Total duration (minutes) and percentage of ischemic periods in ECG monitoring. 30 patients on maintenance hemodialysis were characterized by coronary angiography and echocardiography. CAD = coronary artery disease; LVH = left ventricular hypertrophy.

Since anemia is a well-known factor for provoking or maintaining clinically overt myocardial ischemia in cardiology patients, it is of interest to review the role of renal anemia and the effects of erythropoietin (EPO)-induced recompensation of anemia in dialysis patients with LVH and CAD, which are both characterized by a reduced coronary reserve and episodes of myocardial ischemia. Unfortunately, studies on the impact of anemia recompensation on cardiac prognosis in dialysis patients have not yet been published. Thus, indirect evidence from morphological (echocardiographic) studies and functional studies must be substituted.

LEFT VENTRICULAR HYPERTROPHY

LVH is a frequent finding in patients undergoing chronic hemodialysis or continuous ambulatory peritoneal dialysis, and its prevalence is about 60–70% worldwide. Morphologically, LVH in uremia is characterized by the typical triad of hypertrophied myocytes, deposition of surplus collagen extravasally, and thickening of the media of small intramyocardial arteries. However, in contrast to other conditions such as arterial hypertension (without renal disease), the morphological findings are much more prominent. Experimentally, in five of six nephrectomized rats those histologically detectable findings can be seen as early as 10 days after the operation (3), and in normotensive patients with IgA nephropathy and normal renal function a slight rise of arterial pressure within the still normal range and a simultaneous decrease of the early diastolic blood flow over the mitral valve have been observed (E. Ritz, personal communication), indicating early onset of diastolic dysfunction.

Functionally, it has been well documented in hypertensive subjects that LVH is associated with a reduced coronary reserve (4). In dialysis patients, occurrence of disabling angina in the presence of normal coronaries has been described (5), and Figure 1 illustrates that LVH patients frequently suffer from silent ischemia. In contrast to hypertensive subjects, the background situation of dialysis patients for experiencing an even more pronounced myocardial ischemia is much worse: LVH is frequently more evident with an LV muscle mass exceeding 180 g/m^2.

In analogy to the findings in uremic animals (6) and in biopsies from hypertensive patients (4), it can be assumed that atrophy of myocardial microcirculation is one of the factors responsible for myocardial ischemia. Second, in dialysis patients a prevalence of >70% of arterial hypertension, poorly controlled by drug therapy, is not an infrequent finding, especially during short-duration dialysis therapy (7). An elevated aortic pressure requires an increased LV workload and thereby an augmented myocardial oxygen demand. Furthermore, the frequently reduced aortic distensibility in end-stage renal failure (8) is characterized by an increase of the pulsatile component of arterial pressure with augmented systolic and depressed diastolic pressures. Since myocardial perfusion takes place nearly exclusively during diastole and the level of aortic diastolic pressure is crucial for myocardial perfusion, cardiac ischemia can result from decreased oxygen supply. Third, myocardial oxygen supply can be decreased by an elevated LV diastolic pressure, as usually found in association with LVH in ESRD (9). And, last, anemia can contribute to myocardial ischemia in LVH by a reduction of oxygen carriers and by causing or maintaining a hyperdynamic circulation.

From the multifactorial genesis of myocardial ischemia associated with LVH in ESRD, it can be deduced that elimination or partial correction of one factor—anemia—can only partly normalize myocardial perfusion. On the other hand, anemia per se is one of the factors (among arterial hypertension, a.v. dialysis shunt, intermittent inotropic stimulation by calcium, and possible uremic factors) that can be directly responsible for causing LVH. Silberberg et al. (10) have shown that LV muscle mass is independently correlated with the degree of renal anemia. Again, it becomes obvious that correction of anemia can only partly reverse LVH as long as other factors persist.

The majority of intervention studies in ESRD with rhEPO, in which cautious target hematocrits of up to 35% have been achieved, show a partial regression of LV muscle mass, despite an inhomogeneity of LVH degree, comorbidity, and study duration [recently reviewed by Rademacher and Koch (11)]. As shown by London et al. (12), hematocrit is inversely correlated with LV end-diastolic diameter. Consequently, in most rhEPO interventions the principal effect was on LV end-diastolic dimensions, which normalized. Interventricular septum and LV posterior-wall thickness were affected little if at all. In our study, a relatively homogeneous group of hemodialysis patients with LVH was targeted to a hematocrit of 35% (from 25% originally), and only after 16 months of anemia compensation could a very small reduction of LV posterior-wall thickness be detected (13).

Thus, it may be argued that LVH is not affected at all, since the volumelike effect of normalizing diastole dimensions can be dissociated from the inability to influence LV wall thickness. Histological evidence for a regression of "eccentricity" is absent as is the prognostic meaning. It can be assumed that some of the predisposing factors for myocardial ischemia present in LVH might be influenced by anemia recompensation, although direct data are not available.

In the study of Fellner et al. (14), in which hemodynamic measurements were carefully carried out in the same phase of the interdialytic cycle, recompensation of renal anemia by rhEPO resulted in a significant normalization in two of the three major determinants of myocardial energy demand (heart rate and myocardial contractility) without altering the third (systolic LV load). Exacerbation or de novo development of arterial hypertension could tilt this favorable balance. It therefore remains to be shown whether a regression in this type of LVH by anemia recompensation is also associated with a reduction in cardiac mortality. From the data of Himelman et al. (15), who studied the course of LVH following renal transplantation, the time course of regression of LV muscle mass and associated intermyocardial fibrosis might be different. Clinically, it is therefore of importance to prevent causative factors for the development of LVH as early as possible. In this context, *early* "normalization" of blood pressure, parathyroid function, and anemia in the course of renal insufficiency are of utmost importance.

CORONARY ARTERY DISEASE

Myocardial ischemia by occlusion of large epicardial vessels as occurs in CAD is a well-known phenomenon. However, in dialysis patients, symptomatology is atypical and angina pectoris can be absent in the presence of <90% coronary stenoses (16). The reported incidence of 22% for ischemia heart disease (post-myocardial infarction, post-ACVB, angina) in ESRD patients (17) is probably too low because of silent ischemia and therefore underdiagnosed. Screening by routine angiography in the subgroup of diabetic patients over age 45 revealed a prevalence of 85% of (silent) CAD (18). There is casuistic evidence from cardiology patients that symptomatology of CAD can worsen with evolving anemia, and in anemic ESRD patients relief of anemia and disappearance of ischemic ECG signs have been reported following blood transfusions.

In a study of highly selected ESRD patients with significant CAD and exercise-inducible myocardial ischemia demonstrable on ECG, elevation of hematocrit from 25 to 35% was followed by an increase in maximal physical performance and duration of exercise-stress testing (19). The exercise-load-dependent ST depression was nearly absent, when measured during the 25% hematocrit, indicating less myocardial ischemia. This effect can be explained by an increase in oxygen supply and by the normalization of LV diastolic dimension. Thus, in addition to aspirin, beta-blockers, and ACE inhibitors, maintenance in dialysis patients of a 35% hematocrit target is part of secondary CAD prophylaxis. As for acute coronary syndromes, which originate primarily from nonstenosed artery regions (in angiograms) and can be attributed to de novo occlusion by plaque ruptures (20), there is no information in ESRD patients. It is interesting to speculate that anemia or anemia recompensation by the growth factor EPO could interact with plaque stability.

CONCLUSION

In summary, myocardial ischemia can originate from LVH and CAD independently, albeit in ESRD patients both conditions frequently coexist. The adverse effect of chronic ischemic disease in dialysis patients is mediated by heart failure, which is a strong predictor of earlier death (17). Recompensation of renal anemia by EPO to a target hematocrit of 35% initiates a slow and moderate echocardiographic regression of LVH, primarily by normalizing diastolic dimensions, and increases crucial coronary reserve in CAD. Induction of arterial hypertension by EPO may counteract those effects and should be avoided by appropriate therapy. The current data indicate that a target hematocrit of 35% may be more adequate in dialysis patients with cardiac disease than the commonly used target of 30%. Recompensation of anemia should be initiated as early as possible in the course of renal insufficiency, together with antihypertensive therapy to prevent rather than to reverse LVH. The crucial question, however, is whether EPO therapy, recompensation, or complete disappearance of anemia will improve cardiac prognosis.

REFERENCES

1. Raine AEG, McMahon S, Selwood NH, Wing AJ, Brunner FP. Mortality from myocardial infarction in patients on renal replacement therapy in the UK. Nephrol Dialysis Transplant 1991; 6:902.
2. Rutsky E, Rostand S. The management of coronary artery disease in patients with end-stage renal disease. In: Parfrey PS, Harnett JD, eds. Cardiac Dysfunction in Chronic Uremia. Kluwer Academic Publishers, 1992:231–246.
3. Mall G, Rambauseck M, Neumeister A, Kollmar S, Vetterlein F, Ritz E. Myocardial interstitial fibrosis in experimental uremia: implications for cardiac compliance. Kidney Int 1988; 33:804–811.
4. Schwartzkopff B, Motz W, Frenzel H, Vogt M, Knauer S, Strauer B. Structural and functional alterations of the intramyocardial arterioles in patients with arterial hypertension. Circulation 1993; 88:993–1003.
5. Roig E, Betriu A, Castaner A, Magrina J, Sanz G, Mavarra-Lopez F. Disabling angina pectoris with normal coronary arteries in patients undergoing hemodialysis. Am J Med 1981; 71:437–444.
6. Amann K, Wiest G, Zimmer G, Gretz N, Ritz E, Mall G. Reduced capillary density in the myocardium of uremic rats: a stereological study. Kidney Int 1992; 42:1111–1117.
7. Salem M. Hypertension in the hemodialysis population: a survey of 649 patients. Am J Kidney Dis 1995; 26:461–468.
8. London G, Marchais S, Safer M, et al. Aortic and large artery compliance in end-stage renal failure. Kidney Int 1990; 37:137–142.
9. Kramer W, Wizemann V, Thormann J, Kindler M, Müller K, Schlepper M. Cardiac dysfunction in patients on maintenance hemodialysis: the importance of associated heart diseases in determining alterations of cardiac performance. Contr Nephrol 1986; 52:97–109.
10. Silberberg J, Rahal D, Patton R, Sniderman A. Role of anemia in the pathogenesis of left ventricular hypertrophy in end-stage renal disease. Am J Cardiol 1989; 64:222–224.
11. Rademacher J, Koch KM. Treatment of renal anemia by erythropoietin subscription: the effects on the cardiovascular system. Clin Nephrology 1995; 44(suppl 1):S56–S60.
12. London G, Fabiani F, Marchais S, et al. Uremic cardiomyopathy: an inadequate left ventricular hypertrophy. Kidney Int 1987; 31:973–980.

13. Wizemann V, Schäfer R, Kramer W. Follow up cardiac changes induced by anemia compensation in normotensive hemodialysis patients with left ventricular hypertrophy. Nephron 1993; 64:202–206.
14. Fellner S, Lang R, Neumann A, Korcarz C, Borow K. Cardiovascular consequences of correction of anemia of renal failure with erythropoietin. Kidney Int 1993; 44:1309–1315.
15. Himelman RB, Landzberg JS, Simonson JS, et al. Cardiac consequences of renal transplantation: changes in left ventricular morphology and function. J Am Coll Cardiol 1988; 12:915–923.
16. Hässler R, Höfling B, et al. Koronare Herzkrankheit und Herzklappenerkrankungen bei Patienten mit terminaler Niereninsuffizienz. Deutsche Med Wschr 1987; 112:714–718.
17. Parfrey P, Foley R, Harnett J, Kent G, Murray D, Barre P. Outcome and risk factors of ischemic heart disease in chronic uremia. Kidney Int 1996; 49:1428–1434.
18. Manske C, Thomas W, Wany Y, Wilson R. Screening diabetic transplant candidates for coronary artery disease: identification of a low risk subgroup. Kidney Int 1993; 44:617–627.
19. Wizemann V, Kaufmann J, Kramer W. Effect of erythropoietin on ischemia tolerance in anaemic hemodialysis patients with confirmed coronary artery disease. Nephron 1992; 62:161–165.
20. Fuster V. Lewis A. Common Memorial Lecture. Mechanism leading to myocardial infarction: insights from studies of vascular biology. Circulation 1994; 90:2126–2146.

Index